TAO and the Art of JFDI

Just F**king Do It

By Charlie Mills

Table of Contents

Introduction 3

Chapter 1 - Understanding Procrastination 5

Chapter 2 – The Cost of Waiting 14

Chapter 3: The Power of Action 21

Chapter 4: Shifting Mindset 27

Chapter 5 - Introducing The JFDI Philosophy 32

Chapter 6 – Planning to JFDI 37

Chapter 7 – The Blueprint 41

Chapter 8 – Tools and Techniques 47

Chapter 9 – The Role of Habits 52

Chapter 10 – Surrounding Yourself with Doers 70

Outro 82

Introduction

The modern world, with its unending streams of information and the constant pings of notifications, has created an unforeseen challenge: the paralysis of overthinking. Each day, I watch as countless individuals drown in the possibilities of tomorrow, while today slips through their fingers. The future is bright, but it is marred by the shadow of procrastination. Enter the philosophy of JFDI - Just Fucking Do It.

Overthinking is a modern plague. When faced with the sheer volume of available choices, our mind's natural response is to evaluate each one in minute detail. With the digital age, we're no longer comparing two or three options – we're sometimes grappling with hundreds.

Imagine a library with infinite aisles and countless books. Each book represents an opportunity, an idea, a dream. Now, imagine trying to read the synopsis of each one before deciding which to read first. Overwhelmed? That's how many of us feel every single day.
In the world of entrepreneurship, overthinking looks like endless business plans that never materialise into businesses. It's market analyses so deep that by the time they're done, the market has evolved. As an athlete, the fear of a misstep, the stress over the minutiae of technique, or the anxiety of an upcoming match can often overshadow the pure joy and purpose of the sport. As an author, the obsessing over a character profile, the perfecting of the story arch, the fifth draft of the chapter outline can stretch so long we never actually get a word on the page.

Why We Procrastinate

Take for example my university days, where procrastination was as regular as morning coffee. Late-night study sessions, cramming for exams the day before, and racing against time were the norms. But why? Was it the thrill of the challenge, or was it the fear of facing the vastness of what needed to be done?

Procrastination is a multifaceted beast. For some, it's the fear of inadequacy, for others, it's the overwhelming pressure of potential success. In the world of sports, it might mean delaying training, waiting for the perfect conditions, or pushing back against challenges. In business, it's the waiting for market conditions to be "just right" or seeking endless validations before launching a product.

Unleashing the Power of JFDI

Now, imagine if, during those university days, instead of succumbing to procrastination, I had embraced the JFDI philosophy. How different would things have been? JFDI is more than a call to action. It's a battle cry against inertia. It's the antidote to overthinking.

Every second matters. A millisecond can decide between gold and silver. What if, instead of overanalysing each move, every now and then, we trusted our instincts and just took the plunge?

JFDI doesn't advocate recklessness. Rather, it champions the idea of breaking the initial barrier of inertia, of taking that first step, however imperfect. For in action lies the wisdom and experience no amount of planning can offer. The world's most prominent success stories are not tales of flawless planning but narratives of persistence, of starting, stumbling, learning, and then marching forward with renewed determination.

Remember, the world doesn't reward thinkers; it rewards the doers. And to become a doer, sometimes, you have to JFDI.

Chapter 1 - Understanding Procrastination

Before moving into the actionable steps in this book, it is first important to understand the root causes of our inability to get started. This will be split down between biological, emotional and external triggers. The understanding segments of this book are critical for awareness and pattern recognition to allow you to diagnose these traits and intervene when required.

Biological Roots of Procrastination

Procrastination, often vilified as a sign of laziness or inefficiency, has deeper roots embedded in our evolutionary history. Understanding these roots can shed light on why this behaviour is so prevalent today, even when it seems counterproductive.

Our ancestors lived in an environment vastly different from ours. Their world was defined by immediate dangers: predators lurking in shadows, sudden climatic shifts, or hostile tribes around the corner. This immediacy dictated their behavioural responses.

The Fight or Flight Response: The 'fight or flight' system was a crucial evolutionary development, facilitating immediate reactions to threats. In situations of danger, adrenaline would surge, sharpening senses and preparing the body either to confront the threat (fight) or flee from it (flight). However, this mechanism is geared towards immediate, short-term threats, not long-term projects or tasks.

Modern-day procrastination can be likened to a misfiring of this system. When faced with a task, especially one that feels large or daunting, the brain perceives it as a 'threat'. But instead of a predator, it's the threat of potential failure, effort, or uncertainty. Procrastinating, or 'fleeing' from the task, becomes a form of coping.

Energy Conservation: Life in the wild was unpredictable. Days of abundance were followed by periods of scarcity. In such an environment, it made sense to save energy unless there was a guaranteed immediate benefit. Our ancestors, therefore, evolved to be naturally wary of tasks that didn't promise clear, quick returns.

In today's context, a task like starting a business, writing a book or starting a new exercise regime doesn't promise immediate benefits. Our ancient brain, trying to conserve energy, might resist engaging in such long-term ventures, leading to procrastination.

Brain Structures and Their Roles

The human brain, a product of millions of years of evolution, plays a pivotal role in procrastination.

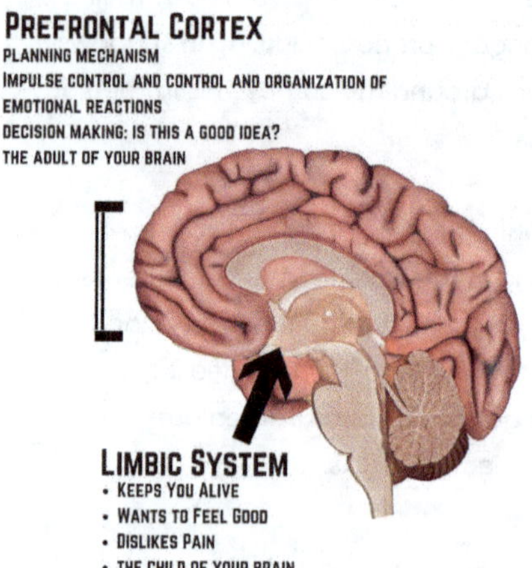

The Limbic System vs. The Prefrontal Cortex:
The limbic system, one of the oldest parts of the brain, governs basic emotions and functions. It's impulsive and seeks immediate pleasure, making it responsible for instinctual reactions, like the 'fight or flight' response.

Contrastingly, the prefrontal cortex, a more recent evolutionary development, is responsible for self-control, planning, decision-making, and understanding consequences. This part of the brain allows us to think about the long-term and suppress impulsive desires.

Procrastination often arises from the tussle between these two. For instance, when deciding whether to work on a project (long-term benefit) or watch a TV show (immediate pleasure), the limbic system's pull towards the latter can overpower the prefrontal cortex's rational arguments.

Genetics and Procrastination

Recent research has hinted at the possibility of a genetic predisposition to procrastination. While the idea is still debated, some studies have found that certain gene variants, particularly those affecting dopamine regulation in the brain, might be linked to a tendency to procrastinate. Dopamine is crucial for motivation, and any imbalance can sway our decision-making processes.

Hormonal Influence

Cortisol, often labelled the 'stress hormone,' has a complex relationship with procrastination. When faced with stress, be it from an impending deadline or the scope of a task, cortisol levels rise. While it's beneficial in short bursts, chronic elevation can lead to fatigue, mood swings, and impaired cognitive functions.

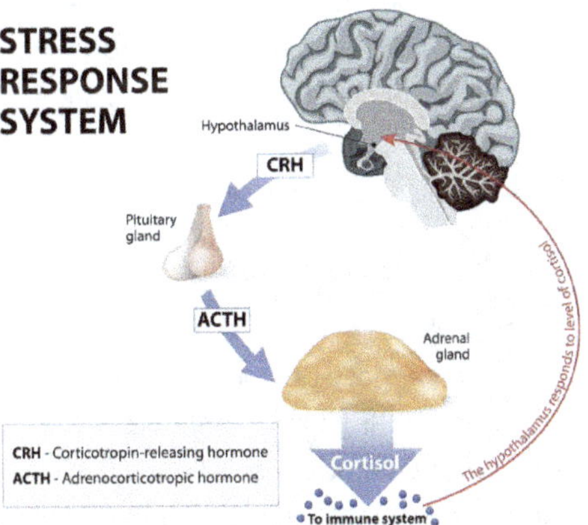

High cortisol levels can make tasks seem even more daunting, pushing one further into the procrastination spiral. On the flip side, the act of procrastination can lead to feelings of guilt and anxiety, further elevating cortisol levels. It becomes a vicious cycle.

The biological roots of procrastination are deep-seated, interwoven with our evolutionary journey. From ancient survival mechanisms to the intricacies of our brain structures and even potential genetic markers, these factors provide context for our modern-day struggles with delay and inaction. Recognizing that procrastination isn't merely a 'lack of willpower' but a complex interplay of evolutionary adaptations can pave the way for compassion and more effective strategies to combat it. Armed with this understanding, we can better harness the power of JFDI, working with our biology rather than against it.

The Emotional Underpinnings of Procrastination

At the intersection of behaviour and emotion lies procrastination, a curious phenomenon where our feelings steer us away from actions that we know are in our best interest. To truly tackle procrastination, we must delve deep into the emotional landscape that underpins it.

1. <u>Fear as a Dominant Driver</u>

Fear of Failure: Perhaps the most cited reason for procrastination is the fear of failure. For many, the thought of not meeting expectations, whether their own or those of others, can be paralyzing. Every delay becomes a shield, protecting them from potential criticism or judgment. In the competitive arenas of sports and business, this fear is amplified. No one wants to be seen as lacking, inadequate, or unprepared.

Fear of Success: Ironically, some are afraid of what might happen if they succeed. Success often brings change – heightened expectations, more responsibilities, and increased scrutiny. For those comfortable in their current state or fearful of the unknown, the idea of succeeding can be as daunting as failing.

Fear of the Unknown: Treading uncharted waters can be intimidating. Whether it's launching a new product, exploring a new training regime, or embarking on a new career, the myriad of unforeseeable challenges can lead to hesitancy. The question "What if?" becomes a formidable barrier.

2. <u>The Weight of Self-Doubt</u>

An internal monologue of doubt can be the most potent deterrent. Questions like "Am I good enough?", "Do I have the expertise?", or "What if there's someone better than me?" can erode confidence. In my athletic pursuits, I've seen incredibly talented individuals second-guess their capabilities, leading them to delay or even abandon their goals. Similarly, in the entrepreneurial world, brilliant minds often grapple with impostor syndrome, feeling they don't belong or fearing they'll be exposed as frauds.

3. <u>The Emotional Burden of Past Experiences</u>

Past experiences, especially those marred by trauma, criticism, or failure, can cast long shadows. A failed venture, a project that didn't get off the ground, or harsh feedback can leave emotional scars. These scars, if not addressed, become triggers for future procrastination. The thought process becomes, "I failed once; what's stopping it from happening again?" It's an emotional defence mechanism — by not starting, one avoids potential pain.

4. <u>Avoidance and Emotional Comfort</u>

Often, procrastination is an act of seeking emotional comfort. When faced with a challenging task, our emotional self yearns for the solace found in easier, more pleasurable activities. Watching a movie, scrolling through social media, or engaging in idle chit-chat offers immediate emotional gratification, a comforting respite from the anxiety or stress of the impending task.

5. <u>Perfectionism and the Pursuit of the Ideal</u>

While perfectionism is often seen as a virtue, it can be a double-edged sword. The relentless pursuit of perfection can lead to an emotional gridlock. The thought of producing something less than perfect becomes emotionally distressing. Perfectionists often grapple with the weight of their own expectations. Every task becomes a reflection of their self-worth, and the fear of producing subpar work leads to endless delays.

The emotional undercurrents of procrastination are deep and multifaceted. It's not merely a matter of laziness or a lack of motivation. Our feelings, past experiences, fears, and doubts all converge to create this behaviour. However, recognising and understanding these emotional triggers is the first step in addressing and overcoming procrastination. In the subsequent chapters, armed with the mantra of JFDI, we'll explore strategies to navigate this emotional maze, ensuring our feelings propel us forward rather than hold us back.

Modern Day Triggers of Procrastination

In an age characterized by technological advancements, constant connectivity, and a flood of information, modern life brings with it a unique set of challenges that amplify our tendencies to procrastinate. While our ancestors had to grapple with survival-based delays, today's procrastination often stems from distractions and overwhelming choices prevalent in our digital age.

1. <u>Overload of Information and Choices</u>

In the past, choices were limited and often clear-cut. Today, the sheer amount of information available at our fingertips, while a boon, often leads to analysis paralysis. Be it choosing a software for a new business, deciding on a workout regime, or even selecting a movie to watch, the multitude of options can be paralyzing. Research indicates that when presented with too many choices, individuals often delay making a decision or avoid it altogether.

2. <u>Instant Gratification and Digital Distractions</u>

Our modern environment is teeming with immediate rewards. Social media platforms, with their infinite scrolls, notifications, and dopamine-driven 'likes', are designed to keep us engaged. Video streaming platforms with auto-playing episodes make it tempting to bingo-watch. Online games, news alerts, and even shopping apps offer quick pleasures with minimal effort. These platforms and their instant rewards often overshadow tasks that require sustained attention and offer delayed gratification.

3. <u>The Comparative World of Social Media</u>

Platforms like Instagram, Facebook, and Twitter have transformed the way we view success. We're constantly bombarded with curated success stories, be it a peer's start-up achievement, a friend's exotic vacation, or even someone's perfect daily routine. These endless streams of others' highlight reels can engender feelings of inadequacy, leading to self-doubt and procrastination. The thought process becomes, "I'll never match up, so why start?"

4. <u>Endless Multitasking</u>

The modern world celebrates multitasking. From juggling emails, meetings, and projects at work to managing social commitments, fitness goals, and personal projects, the drive to do it all has never been more pronounced. However, such multitasking can be overwhelming. The continuous mental switching between tasks can reduce focus, make tasks seem insurmountable, and thereby, increase procrastination.

5. <u>Perfection in the Digital Age</u>

The online world often demands perfection. Be it the perfect Instagram photo, the immaculate blog post, or the flawless video presentation, there's a relentless drive to curate and present the best version of oneself. This obsession with perfection, amplified by digital tools that allow endless tweaking and editing, can become a significant trigger for procrastination.

6. <u>Remote Work and Lack of Physical Accountability</u>

The shift towards remote work, further propelled by global events like the COVID-19 pandemic, brings unique challenges. The lack of a physical office, the absence of colleagues, and a blurred line between personal and professional life can reduce external accountability. Without someone physically checking on progress or without the structure of an office environment, the temptation to delay tasks increases.

Modern-day triggers for procrastination are intricately linked with the very conveniences and advancements that characterize our age. While these tools and platforms offer unparalleled advantages, they also present challenges that require awareness and strategies to overcome. Recognising these triggers is the first step. The subsequent chapters will delve into harnessing the mantra of JFDI to navigate this modern landscape effectively, ensuring that we remain masters of our time and choices.

Chapter 2 – The Cost of Waiting

This book is a call to action. For those who have ideas, but fail to start (or finish) their execution. Therefore, in order to promote action, it's important to understand the consequences of inaction.

Missed Opportunities

Time's Relentless March:
Time, often considered as an abstract entity, is tangible in its consequences. Once passed, it never returns, making its preservation and utilisation paramount. Every moment we procrastinate, potential opportunities fade away into the shadows of the past. In the fast-paced realm of today's world, waiting even a single moment can drastically alter outcomes. Whether it's the fleeting window to launch a start-up in a niche market, a limited-time scholarship offer, or the golden hour for photographers, time-sensitive opportunities abound.

Networking and Building Relationships:
The world, in many ways, functions on relationships. Every event or gathering skipped, every introduction postponed, and every call not returned, can equate to a missed chance at building valuable relationships. In both athletic and entrepreneurial terrains, networking isn't just about expanding contact lists. It's about fostering meaningful partnerships, unearthing mentorship opportunities, or discovering sponsorships that could change the trajectory of one's career. By delaying these engagements, we not only lose the immediate opportunity but potentially countless others that could have sprouted from that one connection.

Windows of Innovation:
Innovation waits for no one. History is peppered with stories of inventions, business ideas, or even creative projects that were conceived by multiple individuals around the same time. What sets apart those who are remembered from those who are forgotten is often a matter of who acted first. Procrastination in such scenarios doesn't just mean missing out; it can mean getting entirely overshadowed.

Personal Growth and Development:
Life offers a myriad of opportunities for personal growth — workshops, courses, training sessions, seminars, and more. Delaying participation or indefinitely postponing such endeavours might seem harmless. Still, over time, these missed chances accumulate into vast gaps in knowledge, skills, or even personal well-being. What could have been a transformative experience or a pivotal moment of insight becomes yet another "what if" in the chronicles of our lives.

Experiences and Memories:
While missed opportunities in professional realms have clear consequences, it's also vital to recognize the intangible losses in our personal lives. Delaying travels, postponing family gatherings, or simply waiting for the "right moment" to pursue a passion can mean missed memories and experiences. Life, in its essence, is a collection of moments, and each one postponed is a page left blank in the narrative of our existence.

Opportunities, both big and small, shape the course of our lives. They are the crossroads leading to various possible futures. In grabbing hold of these chances, we script not just our destinies but also the legacies we leave behind.

The Mental Toll

Every time we succumb to the allure of inaction, we unknowingly levy a tax on our minds. This toll, though intangible, manifests in ways that impact our emotional well-being, mental clarity, and overall zest for life. By diving deep into the psychological repercussions of delay, we can better appreciate the urgency to break free from its shackles.

The Weight of Unfinished Business:
Each task postponed doesn't just vanish. Instead, it lingers, casting a shadow on our psyche. This mental backlog can feel like a weight on our shoulders, leading to a constant undercurrent of anxiety. It's akin to having multiple browser tabs open — each unattended task consumes cognitive resources, leading to mental fatigue and diminished focus on present activities.

Cycle of Guilt and Regret:
One of the most insidious aspects of procrastination is the ensuing cycle of guilt and regret. With every task delayed, guilt creeps in, gnawing at our conscience. Over time, as opportunities slip away, this guilt transforms into regret — a more permanent and poignant emotion that reminisces on what could have been.

Erosion of Self-Trust:
Each time we set a goal and then delay its pursuit, we subtly erode the trust we have in ourselves. This diminishes our self-efficacy, or the belief in our abilities to achieve set goals. Over time, this can lead to a self-fulfilling prophecy, where our doubts breed inaction, and this inaction further reinforces our doubts.

Reinforcing Negative Self-Image:
Procrastination often breeds negative self-talk. Thoughts like "I'm lazy," "I can never get things done," or "I'm a perpetual procrastinator" start to

define our self-image. This negative internal dialogue can be detrimental, affecting not only our self-esteem but also our interactions with others and our outlook on life.

Emotional Exhaustion:
Juggling unfinished tasks and facing the subsequent emotional fallout is exhausting. Over time, the mental strain can lead to burnout, making even simple tasks feel insurmountable. This emotional exhaustion isn't just limited to work or primary pursuits; it bleeds into leisure activities, hobbies, and even interpersonal relationships.

Paralysis by Analysis:
Frequent procrastination, especially when rooted in perfectionism, can lead to overthinking. This "paralysis by analysis" is where one becomes so engrossed in pondering every possible outcome or detail that they become paralyzed, unable to make decisions or take action. This cognitive loop can be mentally draining and is a substantial barrier to productivity and creativity.

The mental toll of inaction is multifaceted and profound. It's not merely about the immediate stress of unfinished tasks but the cumulative impact on our mental health and self-perception. Recognizing these emotional and psychological costs sets the stage for understanding why proactive action — the essence of JFDI — isn't just beneficial but crucial for our mental well-being.

The Time Lost

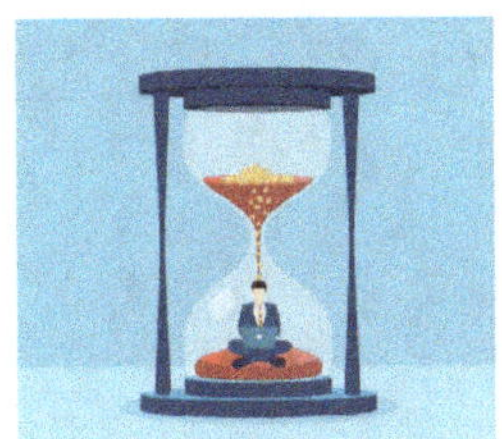

Time is the one resource we cannot regenerate, making its optimal utilisation paramount. When we procrastinate, we're not merely pushing tasks to a later date; we're actively losing moments that could be spent enriching our lives or pursuing our passions. Delving into the intricate tapestry of lost time helps us grasp the imperativeness of seizing the present.

The Compound Effect:
The compound effect emphasises the exponential benefits or repercussions over time. In the context of time lost to procrastination, consider this: if one were to waste just an hour a day, it accumulates to 365 hours in a year — equivalent to over two weeks of continuous activity. Now, imagine the skills that could be honed, the knowledge acquired, or the projects completed in those two weeks.

Every hour spent procrastinating has an opportunity cost. It's the value of the most beneficial activity we forego. For instance, if an entrepreneur delays starting a business, the opportunity cost isn't just the time wasted but potentially the success of that business, the experiences learned, and the impact it might have had on society.

Temporal Illusions:
One of the most insidious aspects of procrastination is the illusion that there's always more time. This mindset creates a false sense of security, making it easy to justify delays. However, with unpredictable events and the ever-evolving nature of life, banking on the future is a perilous gamble.

The Financial Cost

The tendrils of waiting not only snake into our emotional and temporal spheres, but they also burrow deep into our financial health. Understanding the monetary repercussions of delay is critical, especially when we consider finance as a core pillar that supports many of our aspirations and basic needs.

Lost Revenue Opportunities:
For entrepreneurs, professionals, and businesses, time often equates to money. Every project delayed, client not pursued, or product not launched on schedule can represent significant revenue foregone. Especially in markets characterized by high competition, a slight delay can result in a competitor gaining a crucial edge, translating into tangible monetary losses.

Increased Costs:
In the business realm, time affords the luxury of negotiation. Whether it's sealing a deal, sourcing materials, or hiring talent, having the advantage of time often means better rates, terms, or quality. When pressed against the wall due to procrastination, businesses and individuals may have to settle for less favourable conditions, which can have financial ramifications.

Procrastination can lead to situations where rush fees or overtime payments become necessary to meet deadlines. Whether it's a business project, a home repair, or even a last-minute gift purchase, delayed actions often come with inflated price tags. Moreover, postponing essential tasks, like car or home maintenance, can transform minor issues into major, costlier repairs down the line.

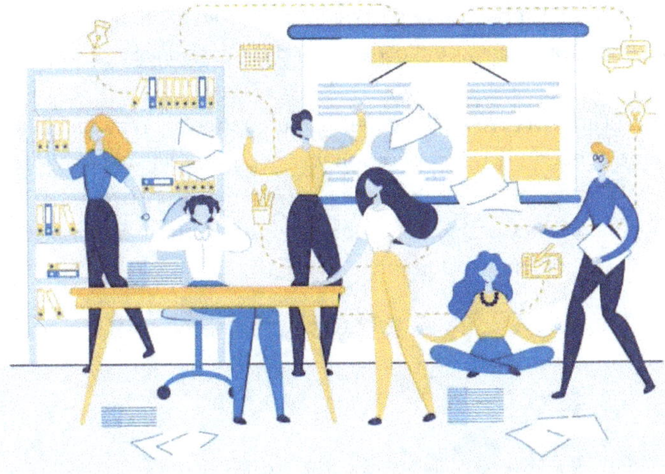

Missed Investment Opportunities:
In the world of finance and investment, timing can be everything. Procrastinating on making an investment or hesitating to capitalize on market opportunities can mean missing out on significant returns. For instance, the difference between investing in a booming stock early versus a week later can be monumental.

Penalties and Late Fees:
One of the more direct financial consequences of procrastination is the accumulation of penalties or late fees. Delaying bill payments, tax submissions, or loan installments can result in hefty fines, higher interest rates, or even legal consequences. Over time, these seemingly small amounts can compound, eating into one's savings. Those of us with tendencies to procrastinate in one area of our life, often do so in others. In my twenties I was guilty of delaying bill payments, not because I couldn't afford it, but because it could wait until tomorrow. That was until I got a court judgement in my name for a menial sum that I could afford to pay 20x over.

Every dollar spent on rectifying the consequences of procrastination is a dollar not invested elsewhere. This not only represents the immediate loss but also the potential future value of that money. Moreover, consistently facing the financial repercussions of delay can strain future budgets, forcing compromises on essential needs or desired luxuries.

The financial impacts are multifaceted and far-reaching. They touch upon both our personal and professional spheres, subtly eroding our financial stability and potential wealth. Recognizing these monetary pitfalls reinforces the urgency of the JFDI philosophy, pushing us to act promptly and safeguard our financial futures.

Chapter 3: The Power of Action

That's the negative part out of the way. Now that we understand why starting is the hardest part, we move into how to take decisive action. How to move from contemplation to concrete steps and learn that getting started is half the battle won.

Momentum: Your New Best Friend

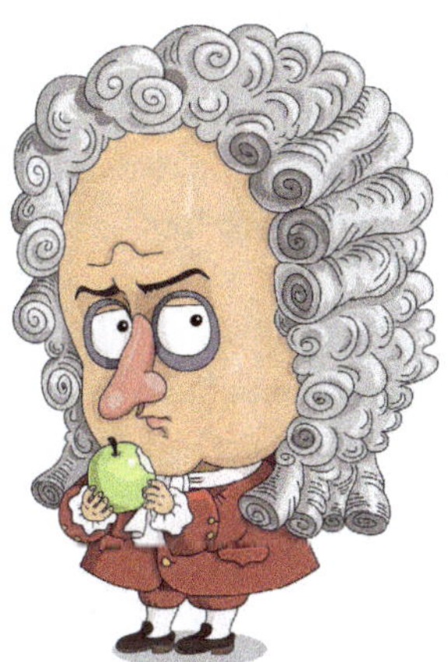

Momentum, often imagined as the unseen force that keeps an object moving, is not just limited to the world of physics. In the realm of personal growth, goals, and endeavours, momentum becomes the silent ally that amplifies our efforts, propelling us forward with a force that can be both unexpected and exhilarating. This section dives deep into understanding momentum's transformative power, illustrating why once you harness it, it becomes an inseparable partner on your journey.

Just as Newton's first law of motion explains that an object in motion stays in motion unless acted upon by an external force, human actions work similarly. Once we overcome the initial resistance and get moving, maintaining that motion becomes considerably easier. The energy required to initiate an action is often significantly greater than what's needed to sustain it.

Imagine a snowball at the top of a hill. Initially, it's small, and starting its descent seems insignificant. But as it rolls down, it gathers more snow, increasing in size and speed. Our actions work similarly. Small, consistent steps can accumulate, leading to substantial progress over time.

As with compound interest in finance, where small, regular investments can lead to significant returns over time, the compounding effect of consistent efforts cannot be underestimated. Every action builds upon the previous one, creating a chain reaction of positive outcomes.

Each time you achieve a task or a milestone, no matter how minor, it sends a positive reinforcement signal to your brain. This boost in confidence makes tackling subsequent tasks seem less daunting, further fueling your drive.

Physical activities, like exercise, release endorphins – our body's natural painkillers that also trigger positive feelings. Similarly, achieving tasks can lead to a sense of euphoria, creating a positive feedback loop that motivates us to achieve even more.

Creating a rhythm and establishing a routine will drive momentum. As you consistently act, this pattern reduces the mental load of initiating tasks, as they become a natural part of your day-to-day life.

Consistent actions provide a sense of predictability in an otherwise chaotic environment. This order can be a source of solace, guiding you through challenges with a clearer mind. As actions are repeated, the initial resistance or inertia diminishes. What once seemed like a challenge becomes second nature, demanding less conscious effort and thought.

The brain is a malleable organ, constantly forming new connections. As you repeatedly perform an action, neural pathways strengthen, making the task easier and more instinctive with each repetition.

Alas, 'an object in motion stays in motion' isn't the reality for anyone in the real world. Even in our journeys, there are moments of stagnation or plateaus. Momentum, cultivated over time, can be the driving force that pushes us through these phases, preventing discouragement and ensuring continuous progress. We lose track? We look over our shoulders and see the results our recent efforts have yielded, be that mental, physical, financial, output. It becomes much easier to jump back on the wagon. To simply 'begin again'.

Momentum is not just a concept; it's a transformative force. By understanding its nuances and consciously harnessing its power, one can navigate the journey from contemplation to realization with more ease and confidence. As the age-old adage goes, "A rolling stone gathers no moss." By fostering momentum, we ensure not only continuous movement but also progress, growth, and eventual success. Embrace momentum; let it be your guiding light, your motivator, and indeed, your new best friend.

Real World Success Stories – Embracing Momentum

Airbnb: From Renting an Air Mattress to Revolutionising Travel

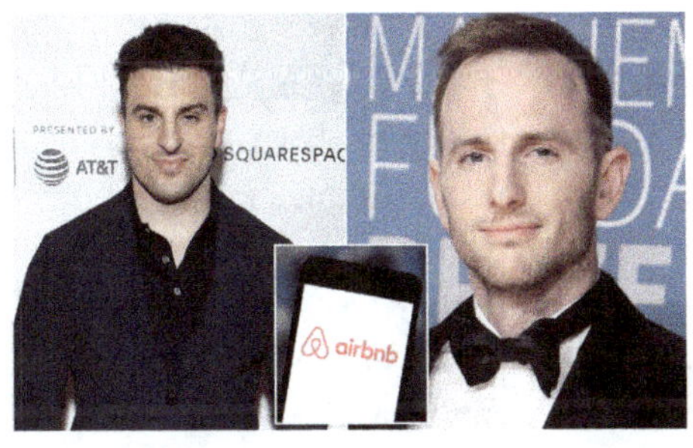

In 2007, roommates Brian Chesky and Joe Gebbia struggled to pay their rent in San Francisco. They decided to turn their living space into a makeshift bed and breakfast for a design conference, offering attendees a place to sleep on air mattresses and serving them breakfast. They created a website, "Air Bed & Breakfast," and had their first guests.

What started as a way to make extra cash turned into a game-changing idea. Together with Nathan Blecharczyk, they launched Airbnb in 2008. However, the journey was fraught with challenges. Initially, they faced skepticism, with investors reluctant to back an idea that involved strangers staying in people's homes. The trio even resorted to selling politically-themed cereal boxes to fund their venture during the 2008 U.S. Presidential election.

The turning point came when they were accepted into Y Combinator, a startup incubator. Here, they redefined their strategy and focused on close-knit communities, like New York, to build momentum. The concept quickly caught on, and soon, the platform expanded globally.

Today, Airbnb has hosted over 800 million guests in more than 220 countries. The company, once dismissed by investors, has transformed the travel and hospitality sector, demonstrating the incredible power of a simple idea combined with relentless perseverance and the momentum of growing demand.

Colonel Sanders: From a Retired Salesman to a Global Fried Chicken Magnate

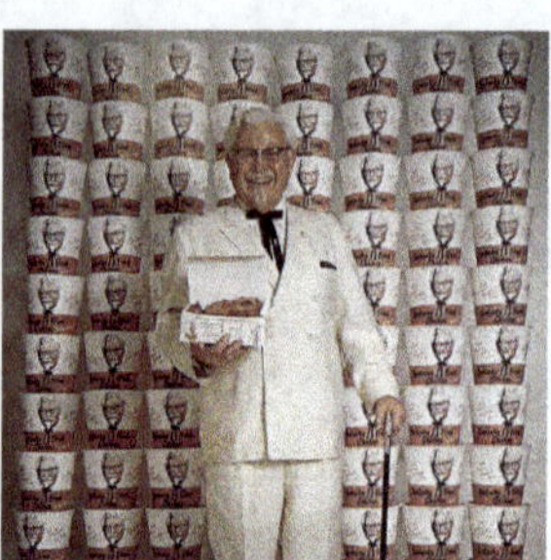

Harland David Sanders, popularly known as Colonel Sanders, experienced a myriad of failures and setbacks throughout his life. At age 40, he ran a service station in Kentucky, serving his specialty: fried chicken. Over time, his local fame grew, leading him to expand his dining space, converting it into a 142-seat restaurant.

However, in the early 1950s, a new interstate was constructed, diverting traffic away from his restaurant and forcing him to sell it at a loss. At 65, with only a $105 monthly social security check, things seemed bleak.

But Sanders was undeterred. Believing in his chicken recipe, he began traveling across the country, cooking batches of chicken for restaurant owners. His proposal was simple: if they liked his chicken, they would enter into a franchise agreement, paying him a nickel for every chicken sold.

He faced over a thousand rejections before finally securing his first franchise in Salt Lake City, Utah. This initial success became the catalyst, and soon, the momentum picked up. By 1964, at the age of 73, Sanders had over 600 franchised outlets for his chicken.

KFC (Kentucky Fried Chicken) has since grown to become one of the largest fast-food chains globally, with more than 24,000 restaurants in over 145 countries. Colonel Sanders' story is a testament to the incredible feats one can achieve when they persistently push forward, allowing the momentum of each small success to pave the way for larger victories.

Sara Blakely: From Selling Fax Machines to Founding Spanx

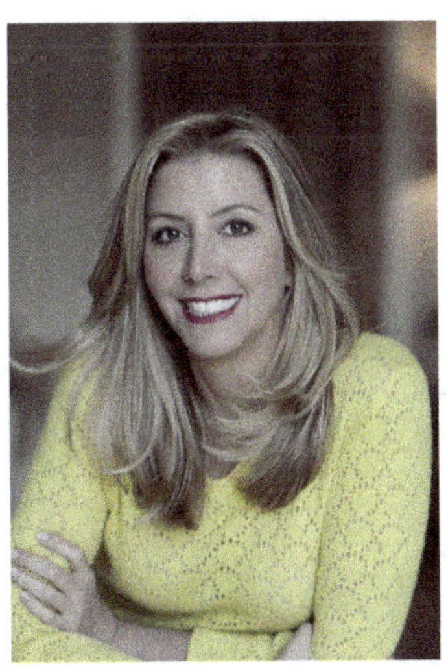

Before she became the youngest self-made female billionaire, Sara Blakely was hustling door-to-door, selling fax machines. It was during these days of corporate sales that she confronted a small problem that would lead to a billion-dollar solution. Wanting to wear white pants to a party but not having the right undergarment that didn't show visible lines or made her feel constricted, Sara took a pair of scissors and cut the feet off her control top pantyhose. The result? A smoother silhouette without any of the constraints.

This moment was the seed for Spanx. However, turning this idea into a product wasn't easy. Blakely faced a slew of rejections, with many hosiery mills unwilling to take a chance on her prototype. Undeterred, she relentlessly pursued her vision. When she finally found a mill owner in North Carolina willing to help her make her product, she spent the next two years patenting her idea and perfecting the prototype.

With savings of $5,000, Blakely launched Spanx in 2000. Rather than spending on traditional advertising, she relied on word of mouth, sending her product to celebrities and appearing on Oprah's television show where Spanx was listed as one of Oprah's "Favorite Things". The endorsement proved a pivotal moment, and the momentum surged. Within its first year, Spanx made $4 million in sales, followed by $10 million in its second year.

Blakely's tenacity combined with her knack for grassroots marketing helped Spanx become a household name. Today, Spanx offers a wide range of undergarments, activewear, and swimwear, and Sara Blakely's story stands as a testament to the power of a simple idea, unshakeable belief, and the momentum that results from sheer persistence.

Chapter 4 – Shifting Mindset

<u>The Power of Imperfection</u>

Embracing imperfection doesn't mean that we advocate for mediocrity or lack of effort. Instead, it's a recognition of our humanity, an acceptance that making mistakes, facing failures, and having flaws are integral parts of our journey.

When we accept imperfection, we foster creativity. Perfection often confines us within rigid boundaries. When we're not constantly worrying about making mistakes, our minds are free to explore, innovate, and think outside the box.

It also helps build resilience. Every setback or mistake offers a lesson. By facing these challenges head-on, we develop a resilient spirit, learning to bounce back and adapt with newfound wisdom.

Finally, it also cultivates authenticity. We are human, and imperfection keeps us genuine. It helps us stay true to ourselves, fostering deeper connections with others who recognise and relate to our shared human experience.

Practical Steps to Embrace Imperfection:

1. Reflect on Past Mistakes: Instead of shying away from past errors, embrace them. Reflect on the lessons they've imparted and how they've moulded your current self.

2. Set Realistic Expectations: Aim for progress, not perfection. Understand that growth is incremental and celebrate small victories along the way.

3. Seek Feedback: Engage with trusted peers or mentors, friends or family, who can provide constructive criticism. Their perspectives can help you identify areas for growth while also highlighting your strengths.

4. Practice Self-compassion: Be kind to yourself. Understand that every individual, no matter how accomplished, has faced setbacks and made mistakes. It's these very experiences that add depth and dimension to our character.

Embracing imperfection is a liberating experience. It allows us to break free from the self-imposed chains of unrealistic expectations and grants us the freedom to pursue our passions without constant self-judgment. By acknowledging our imperfections and viewing them as strengths rather than weaknesses, we position ourselves for genuine growth, deeper connections, and a richer, more fulfilling life journey.

Growth vs Fixed Mindset

Every individual's outlook towards abilities and talents can largely be traced back to their upbringing, early experiences, and societal influences. From a young age, we're often categorized: "She's naturally good at math," "He's a born artist," or "She just doesn't have a knack for languages." These labels, whether intended or not, plant seeds that later grow into our beliefs about our capabilities.

Psychologist Dr Carol Dweck, through her extensive research at Stanford University, shed light on two primary mindsets that shape our perspective and approach towards challenges:

1. *Fixed Mindset:* Individuals with a fixed mindset believe that their talents and abilities are innate and unchangeable. They see

challenges as threats, often avoiding them to not risk appearing less capable. Failures or setbacks are seen not as opportunities for growth but as direct reflections of their abilities. This mindset can lead to avoiding new experiences due to fear of failure or being judged.

2. **Growth Mindset:** In contrast, those with a growth mindset believe that abilities can be developed through effort, training, and perseverance. They view challenges as opportunities to expand their horizons and grow. Setbacks or mistakes are not seen as failures but as valuable feedback, crucial for learning and improvement. This perspective fosters resilience, a love for learning, and a more proactive approach to challenges.

The mindset with which we approach life doesn't just determine our willingness to take on challenges; it influences our overall well-being, satisfaction, and relationships. Here's how:

1. **Resilience**: With a growth mindset, failures become information – feedback loops that guide us toward better approaches. This perspective helps individuals bounce back from setbacks more quickly and with a more positive outlook.

2. **Long-term Achievement**: A growth mindset promotes continuous learning and effort, often leading to greater long-term achievements. Conversely, a fixed mindset may achieve early success but can struggle with adaptability in the face of change or challenges.

3. **Enhanced Relationships**: Individuals with a growth mindset are more likely to foster positive relationships. Their perspective on personal growth often translates into understanding, patience, and a willingness to work through interpersonal challenges.

<u>**Cultivating a Growth Mindset**</u>

Shifting from a fixed to a growth mindset requires conscious effort, but the rewards are manifold. Here are some strategies:

1. **Embrace Challenges**: Instead of shying away from new experiences, actively seek them out. See them as opportunities to learn and grow.

2. **Reframe Failures**: Start viewing setbacks as feedback. Analyse what went wrong, adjust, and move forward with newfound knowledge.

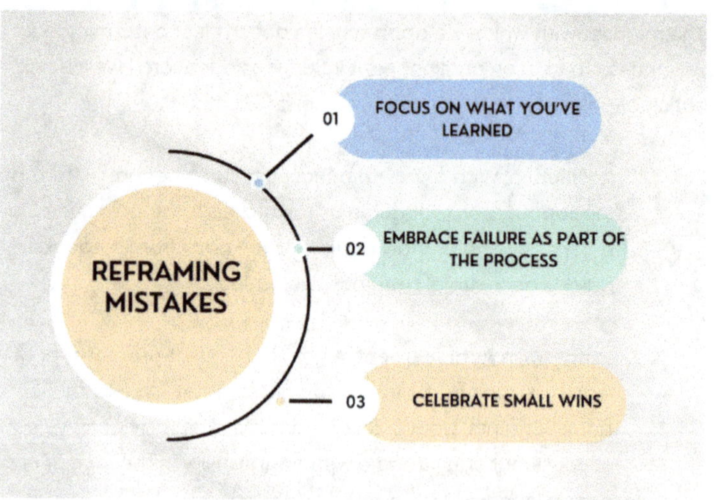

3. **Celebrate Effort Over Outcome**: Praise and reward effort, strategy, focus, perseverance, and improvement. Recognise the process rather than the result.

4. **Continuous Learning**: Cultivate a love for learning. Engage in new courses, read widely, and surround yourself with people who encourage growth.

5. **Mindful Affirmations**: Use affirmations that promote a growth mindset like, "I am capable of learning and growing," or "Challenges help me become better."

Whilst our early experiences and upbringing may influence our initial mindsets, it's essential to understand that mindsets are malleable. With conscious effort, self-awareness, and a genuine desire for growth, anyone can shift from a fixed to a growth perspective. Embracing a growth mindset not only elevates our personal and professional trajectories but also enriches our life experiences, paving the way for a more fulfilling and impactful life journey.

Chapter 5 - Introducing The JFDI Philosophy

JFDI, "Just Fucking Do It", is more than just a catchy phrase; it's a powerful philosophy that challenges the status quo of overthinking, hesitation, and fear. In its raw essence, JFDI is a call to action, urging individuals to leap into the unknown, to make decisions, to start, and to trust in the process.

In the fast-paced age of start-ups, digital advancements, and global entrepreneurship, the idea of "perfect timing" has become obsolete. Traditional methods of planning every step, waiting for the right moment, and endless contemplation have been overthrown by the brave, the bold, and those willing to take risks. JFDI was born from this very evolution, representing a cultural shift towards immediate action, learning from experience, and iterating on the go.

Why JFDI Resonates

1. Combats Analysis Paralysis: In a world saturated with information and choices, many are trapped in the endless cycle of over-analysing situations. JFDI cuts through this noise, advocating for decisive action.

2. Fosters Authentic Learning: There's a profound difference between theoretical knowledge and experiential learning. We promotes the latter, pushing individuals to learn from real-world experiences.

3. Breaks the Fear Barrier: As we've learned, fear of failure, judgment, or the unknown can be paralysing. The JFDI mindset reframes these fears, emphasising the importance of the journey over the destination.

Principles for Implementation

1. **Start Small**: You don't need to make life-altering decisions immediately. Begin with smaller tasks or projects, build confidence, and then tackle bigger challenges with the JFDI mindset.

2. **Trust Your Intuition**: While it's essential to be informed, sometimes our gut feeling or intuition guides us best. Learn to trust this inner voice.

3. **Set a Timer**: For tasks or decisions you've been postponing, set a timer for a specific period (say 5 minutes or an hour). Commit to acting once the timer goes off.

4. **Reflect and Iterate**: JFDI doesn't mean disregarding consequences. After taking action, take the time to reflect, learn from the outcomes, and make necessary adjustments for the future.

5. **Surround Yourself with Doers**: Being around like-minded individuals who embody the JFDI spirit can be incredibly motivating. They not only inspire but also hold you accountable.

While JFDI is a potent philosophy, it's essential to understand its limitations. Blind action without any foresight can lead to unnecessary challenges. The idea is not to bypass planning entirely but to strike a balance, ensuring that planning doesn't become a tool for procrastination.

It is also important to redefine what we mean by 'success'. Success is subjective, and relative. Instead of benchmarking against societal standards or others' achievements, define what success really means for you.

When transitioning to the JFDI mindset, there will inevitably be "what ifs". What if I fail? What if it's not perfect? What if they judge? If not managed properly, these can spiral and be paralysing. I am going to share with you some effective ways to navigate these:

1. **Rationalise the Worst-Case Scenario**: Often, when we objectively assess the worst that can happen, we realise it's not as daunting as our minds made it out to be. Failure is often a better outcome than the feeling of not trying. Remember, the only way to mastery is to first be shit!

2. **Visualise Success**: Channel energy into visualising positive outcomes. Not in a heeby-jeeby woo-woo way, take the time to reflect and imagine the success of your actions. This boosts your confidence and prepares the mind and body to achieve desired results.

3. **Use Action as an Antidote**: The more we dwell, the larger our fears grow. Dive into action, even the smallest step, to break the cycle of overthinking and anxiety.

Seeking Support

Above all, one thing I wanted to stress the most in this chapter is the importance of the willingness to seek support. In introducing JFDI, we must look beneath the surface, at the foundational support.

While the JFDI philosophy urges us to take charge and act, it's crucial to acknowledge that seeking support doesn't equate to weakness. Instead, it's a sign of strength, showing recognition of one's areas of growth and a desire for enhancement. Harnessing external support can greatly accelerate our journey of overcoming fears.

Before we step into support models, it's important to note that not all methods of support will be suitable for all individuals. For example, someone working two jobs to make ends meet won't be going to any workshops or retreats, but they will find solace in free online communities of like minded people and support groups. The goal here is to suggest something for everyone, not everything for everyone.

1. **Mentors and Role Models:** These are individuals who've treaded the path you're venturing onto. They provide:
   - *Guidance*: A mentor can help you navigate challenges, offering solutions from their reservoir of experiences.
   - *Perspective*: They present a broader view, helping you see beyond immediate obstacles.
   - *Reassurance*: Knowing someone has overcome similar barriers can boost confidence and diminish fears.

2. **Therapeutic Interventions**: This goes beyond traditional therapy. It encompasses:
   - *Professional Counselling*: For those with deep-seated fears, professional help can offer coping mechanisms, techniques, and healing.
   - *Life Coaches*: These individuals provide structured guidance, helping align personal and professional goals, and assisting in breaking down barriers.
   - *Workshops & Retreats*: Immersive experiences can offer both learning and healing. They foster personal growth and equip individuals with tools to tackle fears.

3. **Community and Peer Support**: Never underestimate the power of collective strength.
   - *Support Groups*: Safe spaces where individuals share fears, challenges, and success stories. Such groups provide solace and encouragement.

- *Mastermind Groups*: Peer-driven, these groups offer brainstorming, education, and mutual support in a respectful and challenging environment.
- *Networking Events*: Meeting and connecting with like-minded individuals can not only provide support but also open doors to opportunities that help bypass or overcome fears.

Harnessing Digital Support

In the age of technology, support isn't just a physical entity. Value can be found in many places, sometimes those least expected. For example:

- *Online Forums & Communities*: Websites like Reddit and niche-specific forums are treasure troves of experiences, advice, and support.
- *Webinars & Online Courses*: Educational platforms like Coursera, Udemy, and MasterClass offer courses on personal growth, fear management, and skill enhancement.
- *Podcasts & Blogs*: Real-life stories, expert interviews, and motivational content can provide daily doses of inspiration and guidance.

The key is to recognise which support systems resonate most with your journey. Interact, engage, attend sessions if applicable. Participate in discussions and seek advice and feedback. Offer support when others seek it. This not only reinforces your learnings but also strengthens your position within the community.

Chapter 6 – Planning to JFDI

Aiming to "just fucking do it" doesn't mean diving headfirst without a sense of direction. Proper planning is not the enemy of action; in fact, it can be its greatest ally. This chapter will guide you on striking the right balance between meticulous preparation and vigorous execution, ensuring that your determination to act is met with the best possible outcomes.

The Necessity of Planning

In a world increasingly driven by the "hustle culture," where speed and agility are lauded, it's tempting to dismiss planning as a slow, old-fashioned approach. But those who have achieved lasting success know the indispensable value of planning. Let's delve deeper into why planning remains crucial in any undertaking, and how it complements the JFDI philosophy.

<u>Vision: The Compass of Success</u>

Direction and Purpose: Embarking on a journey without knowing the destination is like sailing a ship without a compass. Planning provides clarity on where you want to go and why. It defines the mission and purpose of your endeavour.

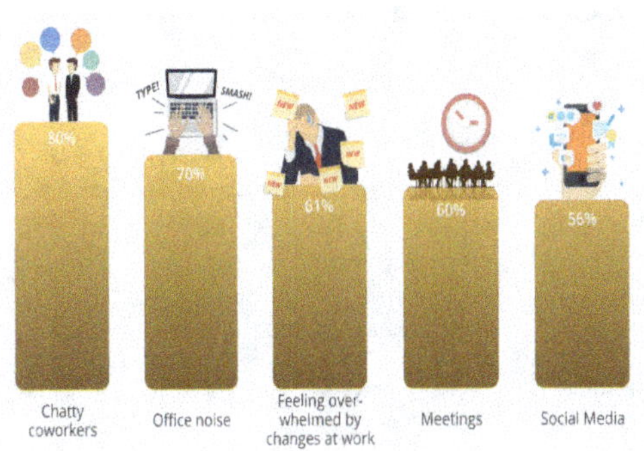

Filtering Distractions: In a world brimming with opportunities and distractions, a clear vision ensures you remain undeterred by the noise, focusing only on what aligns with your ultimate goal.

Inspiration and Drive: A defined vision serves as a constant source of motivation. During challenging times, revisiting this vision can reignite passion and determination.

<u>Efficiency: Maximising Your Resources</u>

Roadmap to the Goal: Think of planning as creating a GPS route. It shows the most efficient path, highlights potential roadblocks, and even provides alternative routes when faced with obstacles.

Conserving Resources: Without a plan, resources—be it time, money, or energy—can be wasted on unfruitful tasks. Planning ensures every action taken contributes to the larger goal, avoiding unnecessary detours or dead-ends.

Enhanced Productivity: When you know the steps to take, the process becomes streamlined. Efficiency reduces the risk of burnout and ensures that you're operating at peak productivity.

<u>Motivation: The Fuel for the Journey</u>

Milestones and Checkpoints: Breaking down the plan into smaller milestones gives tangible points of progress. Celebrating these mini victories can offer motivation boosts, propelling you forward with renewed vigour.

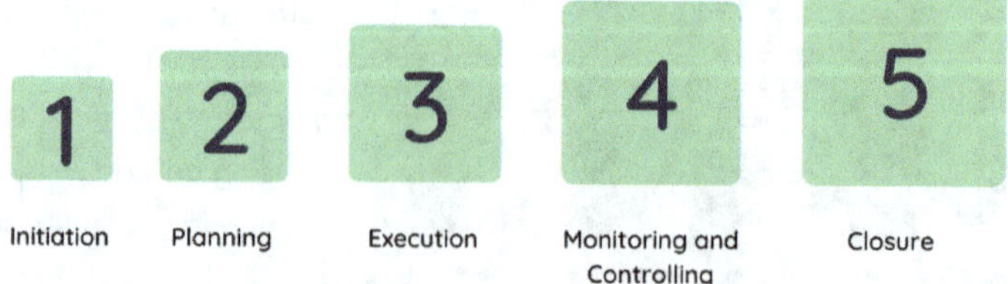

Accountability: A plan serves as a commitment, a promise you make to yourself. It holds you accountable, ensuring that you stay true to your objectives and responsibilities.

<u>Risk Management</u>

Anticipation and Preparation: Planning enables you to foresee potential challenges and devise strategies to tackle or mitigate them. This proactive approach reduces last-minute scrambles and panic.

Contingency Routes: No journey is without its unexpected hurdles. With a plan, you're better equipped to handle unforeseen setbacks, having already considered backup routes and alternative strategies.

Resource Allocation: Knowing potential risks allows you to allocate resources where they're most needed, ensuring that you're not left unprepared when challenges arise.

Planning, in essence, is the foundation upon which the edifice of your dreams is built. It ensures stability, provides direction, and maximises efficiency. While the world may romanticise the idea of spontaneous, unplanned success, the reality is that most triumphs are a product of meticulous planning fused with relentless execution. Embrace planning as a trusted ally in your JFDI journey.

Planning is doing it. The key is to avoid the aforementioned analysis paralysis. Come to your conclusions and move forwards. Perfection is not the goal here. Plan to enable you to make decisions, not to spread doubt in your decision-making process.

Another key thing to avoid is losing flexibility through planning. You must still be able to adapt and be creative, therefore your framework does not need to be over detailed and rigid. JFDI means also being able to think on the fly.

Chapter 7 – The Blueprint

Amid the vast expanse of methodologies, strategies, and planning techniques, the JFDI blueprint emerges as a beacon for those who desire tangible results without getting mired in the quicksand of over-analysis. This blueprint doesn't diminish the value of planning but rather champions a dynamic approach, ensuring that action remains at the forefront. Let's dive into the core tenets of this powerful framework.

The 10 Commandments

1. Keep the End in Mind

Clear Objectives: Begin with a crystallised vision. What do you want to achieve? By when? Strip away the fluff and pinpoint your main goals. These should be concise, specific, and easily understood at a glance.

Visual Aids: Create visual representations of your goals. Vision boards, charts, or even simple post-it notes can serve as daily reminders and motivators, keeping your objectives top of mind.

2. Break It Down

Milestones Over Marathons: Divide the journey into bite-sized milestones. This not only makes the process more digestible but also offers opportunities to celebrate mini victories along the way.

Task Prioritization: Understand the difference between urgent and important. Focus on high-impact activities that drive you closer to your goal, while ensuring urgent tasks don't divert you from the main path.

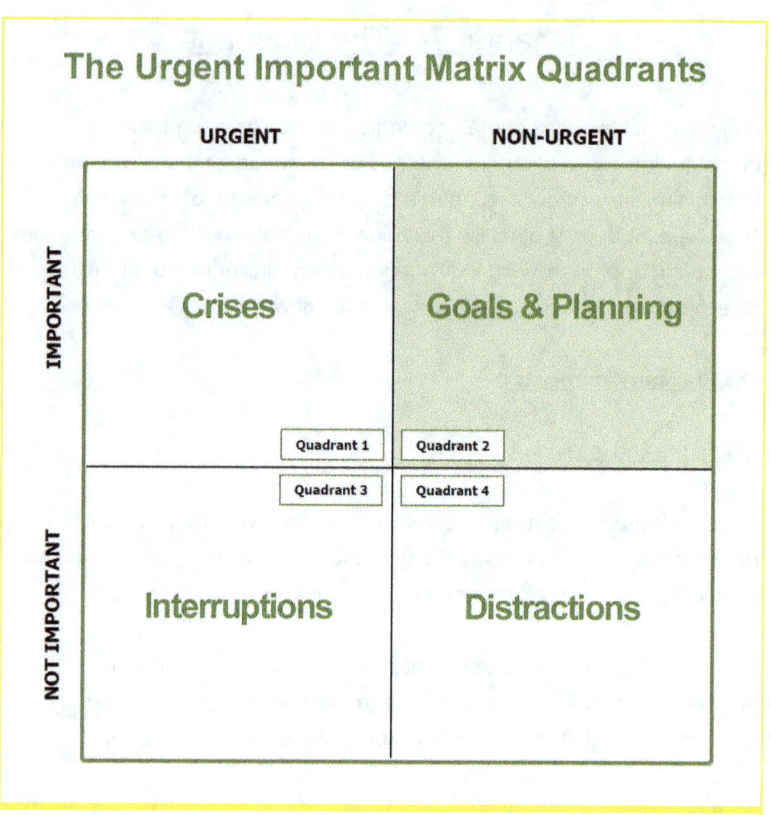

This simple quadrant method allows you to rapidly identify the priority of your tasks. I draw this up at my desk at the beginning each day.

3. Time Management

Set Deadlines: Even if they're self-imposed, deadlines create a sense of commitment. They counteract the human tendency to delay and instil a sense of urgency.

The Power of the Pomodoro: Use techniques like the Pomodoro method, where focused work intervals are interspersed with short breaks. Such techniques harness the brain's capacity for short, intense focus while also offering recuperation.

WHAT IS THE POMODORO TECHNIQUE?

A method for staying focused and mentally fresh

STEP 1		Pick a task
STEP 2		Set a 25-minute timer
STEP 3		Work on your task until the time is up
STEP 4		Take a 5 minute break
STEP 5		Every 4 pomodoros, take a longer 15-30 minute break

4. Embrace Feedback Loops

Regular Reviews: Allocate weekly or monthly review periods to evaluate progress. What's working? What's not? Adjust accordingly. It's about course-correction, not perfection.

Seek External Perspectives: Sometimes, we're too close to a project to see its flaws or potential. Regular feedback from trusted peers or mentors can provide invaluable insights.

5. Guard Against Distractions

Distraction-free Zones: Cultivate environments conducive to work. Whether it's a specific room, a coffee shop, or noise-cancelling headphones, identify and utilize what helps you focus.

Technology Truces: Allocate specific times for emails, social media, and other potential distractions. Apps like "Forest" or "Freedom" can assist in maintaining digital discipline. We are all susceptible to the draw of social media, it has some of the best minds working against us, stealing our attention. When I find myself in a slump of automatically reaching for my phone instead of focusing, I use a KSafe.

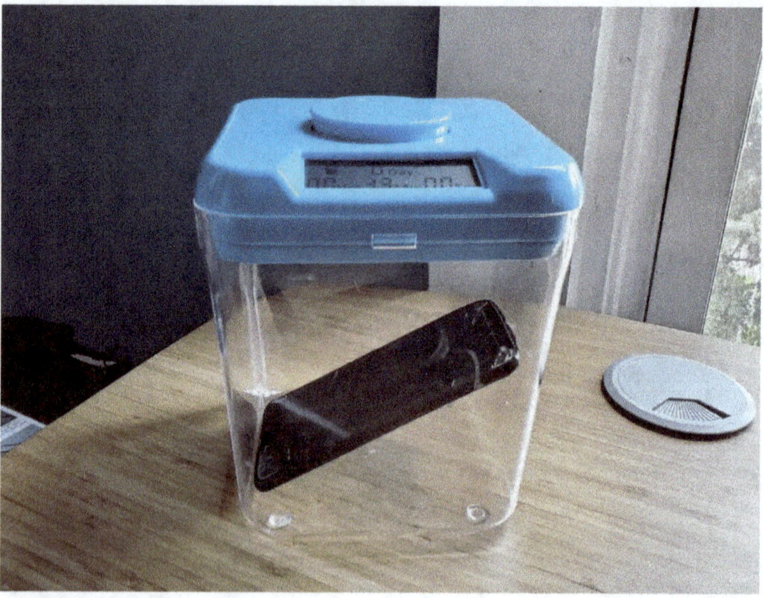

You select a time period, drop your phone in, and you can't have it back until time is up. Simple but effective.

6. Celebrate and Reflect

Reward Mechanisms: Establish a reward system for when milestones are reached. Whether it's a treat, a day off, or a fun activity, let it serve as motivation.

Reflection: Regularly take a step back to reflect on the journey. What have you learned? What can be improved? This ensures continuous growth and avoids stagnation.

7. Remain Agile

Flexibility: While the blueprint provides a structure, remain open to adjustments. If a method isn't working, pivot. Adaptability is a hallmark of the JFDI philosophy.

Iterative Approach: Rather than aiming for one massive launch or completion, adopt an iterative approach. Release versions, gather feedback, refine, and re-release. This ensures continuous progress and improvement.

8. Allocate Resources

Be realistic: Determine what you need in terms of time, money, and other resources. Be realistic in your allocations. An overestimation is better than running short further down the line.

Time: If you plan to go solo in your endeavour, and have cash constraints, understand that the trade-off is time. It's a great motivator for a venture to fly solo, but make sure you understand the time vs resource tradeoff.

<u>9. Prioritise Execution</u>

Action: Once you have a rough plan, dive into action. Remember, the plan is not set in stone, it adapts and evolves.

False starts: Similarly, don't be deterred by a few false starts in your endeavour. This is natural and more often the case than not. You'll be hard stretched to find a success story that doesn't include some major setbacks. Most of which are at the front end.

<u>10. JFDI!</u>

The JFDI blueprint isn't about abandoning planning but refining it to serve action. It's a dynamic, living guide that evolves with your journey. Its essence lies in its adaptability and unwavering focus on forward motion. Embrace it, personalise it, and watch as your endeavours transform from mere ideas into tangible realities.

Chapter 8 – Tools and Techniques

 The JFDI philosophy emphasises action over endless preparation.
However, for action to be impactful, it needs direction. This is where
effective planning tools and techniques come into play. By leveraging
these resources, you can streamline your process, maintain clarity, and
most importantly, drive forward with purpose. Let's explore some of the
most effective tools and techniques to elevate your JFDI journey.

The named tools in this chapter are simply examples of each type and
there are a plethora of alternatives. These are the versions I have used
personally and found valuable. No paid sponsorships, no links, no referrals.

1. Digital Task Managers

Trello: A visual tool that employs a board-card system, enabling users to
move tasks through various stages. With integrations, customizable
boards, and collaboration features, it's great for both individuals and
teams. A personalise favourite for work and personal tasks.

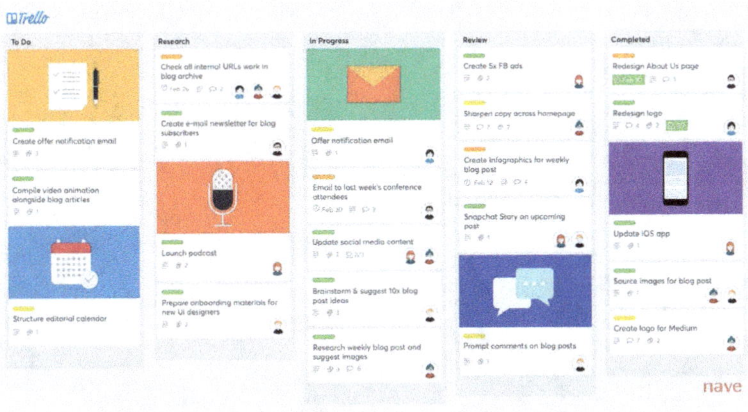

Todoist: A straightforward task management tool, Todoist allows users to create daily to-do lists, set reminders, and categorise tasks with priorities.

2. Time Blocking Techniques

Google Calendar or Microsoft Outlook: It seems simply and basic, but it can be powerful. Use these digital calendars to allocate specific blocks of time for particular tasks. By visually seeing your day, week, or month planned out, you'll be more inclined to stick to the agenda.

The Pomodoro Technique: This method involves working in bursts of intense focus (usually 25 minutes), followed by short breaks. Over time, this can enhance productivity and maintain mental sharpness.

3. Mind Mapping Tools

MindMeister: An intuitive online mind mapping tool that allows for brainstorming sessions, project planning, and visual organisation of complex ideas.

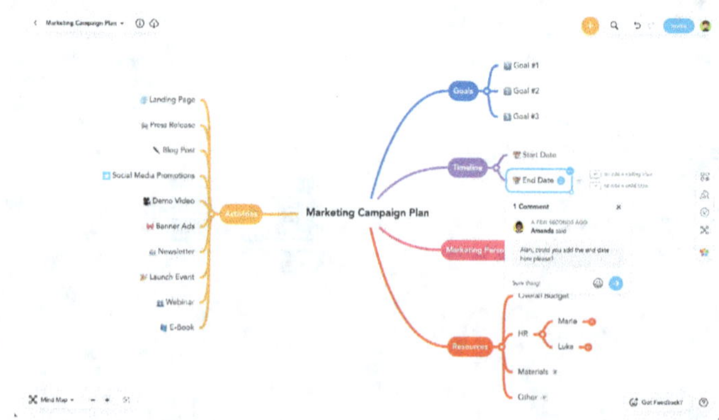

XMind: This software helps in creating intricate mind maps, allowing users to visualize workflows, brainstorm, or structure concepts.

4. Journaling and Note-taking Apps

Evernote: More than a note-taking app, Evernote allows users to capture ideas, save online articles, and collaborate on notes with others.

OneNote: Microsoft's digital notebook where you can jot down ideas, keep meeting minutes, or draft plans. The ability to draw, type, or add images makes it versatile.

5. Goal-setting Frameworks

SMART Goals: This technique emphasises setting goals that are Specific, Measurable, Achievable, Relevant, and Time-bound. It adds clarity and accountability to objectives.

OKRs (Objectives and Key Results): Popularised by companies like Google, OKRs help organisations and individuals align their goals with measurable results, ensuring everyone is moving in the right direction.

Objectives	Key results
Should be ambitious, clearly defined, qualitative and set within a specific time frame.	Should be difficult but achievable.
Need to be communicated and understood by all employees and stakeholders.	Should be able to be objectively and regularly assessed.
Should be flexible and reviewed regularly.	Can be based on KPIs such as growth, performance, revenue and engagement.

6. Collaborative Platforms

Slack: A communication platform that allows teams to chat in real-time, share files, and integrate with numerous other tools, ensuring everyone stays on the same page.

Asana: A comprehensive project management tool. With task assignments, timelines, and project stages, it helps teams stay aligned and aware of project statuses.

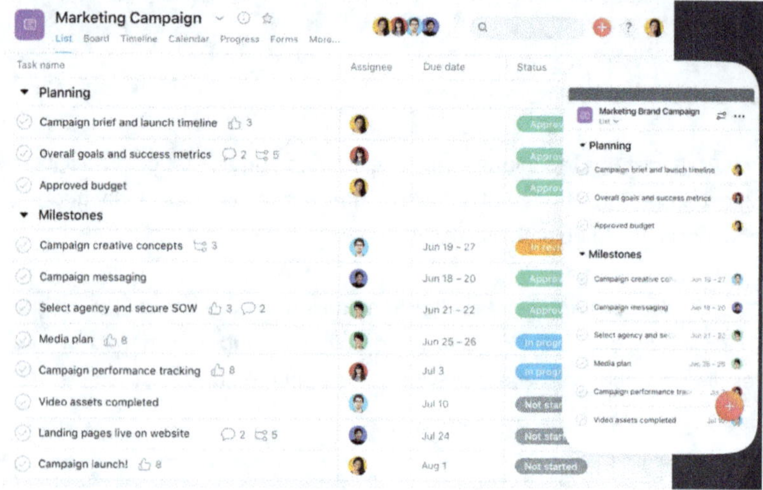

7. Focus Enhancers

Forest App: This app gamifies focus. Plant a tree when starting a task, and if you remain focused, the tree grows. If you get distracted, the tree withers.

Freedom: Block distracting websites and apps for specific periods, helping maintain focus during work sessions.

K-Safe: A physical safe with a timer. You place your phone in the safe, set the amount of time you wish to keep it there and the commitment is made. I've found this to be the most effective, and they are relatively cheap.

8. Regular Review Systems

Weekly Review Rituals: Allocate a specific time each week to review tasks accomplished, goals met, and what needs adjustment. This consistent reflection ensures alignment with objectives.

Quarterly Check-ins: A more in-depth review process that assesses progress on broader goals, ensuring long-term objectives remain in focus.

The JFDI philosophy champions action, and the right tools and techniques supercharge this action. They provide the necessary structure, clarity, and efficiency, ensuring that when you leap into action, it's both informed and impactful. Familiarize yourself with these resources, adapt them to your unique needs, and you'll find that the journey from thought to action becomes a seamless, powerful transition.

Chapter 9 – The Role of Habits

In the journey of actualising our goals and realising our ambitions, the mantra of JFDI plays a central role. However, the sustainability of this spirited drive hinges on one crucial element: habits. These small consistent actions compound over time and produce substantial results. In this chapter we will explore the influence of habits, how they're formed, and how to tailor them to propel us toward success.

The Science of Habits

Delving into the science of habits, it becomes evident that these patterns of behaviour aren't merely accidental repetitions or mindless routines. They are deeply rooted in our neurobiology, shaped by evolutionary mechanisms to increase efficiency and save cognitive energy.

1. Neurological Foundations of Habits

Neuroplasticity: At its essence, the brain is malleable, with its ability to reorganise itself by forming new neural connections. This plastic nature ensures that repetitive behaviours strengthen neural pathways, making subsequent repetitions easier and more automatic. Over time, these reinforced actions morph into habits.

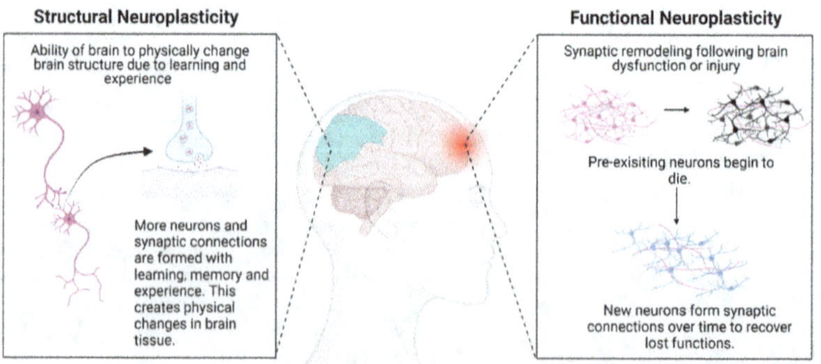

Basal Ganglia: This ancient part of the brain plays a pivotal role in the formation and retention of habits. While the prefrontal cortex is active when we're learning a task (say, tying shoelaces), over repetition, the basal ganglia take over, making the process automatic and freeing up the prefrontal cortex.

Dopamine and Reward Circuits: Habits aren't solely about repetition; they're also about reward. When a behaviour results in a positive outcome, dopamine—a neurotransmitter associated with pleasure and reward—is released. This reinforces the behaviour, making it more likely to be repeated.

2. The Habit Loop

Cue: Every habit begins with a cue or trigger. It's an event that initiates the habitual behaviour. This could be external, like the chime of a notification prompting you to check your phone, or internal, such as a feeling of stress leading to nail-biting.

Routine: This is the core action or behaviour—the habit itself. It's what ensues post-cue: checking the phone or biting the nails, in the examples.

Reward: The culmination of the loop, the reward is the positive feedback or outcome received from the behaviour. It's the dopamine hit from social media likes or the temporary relief from stress through nail-biting. This reward reinforces the behaviour, strengthening its recurrence.

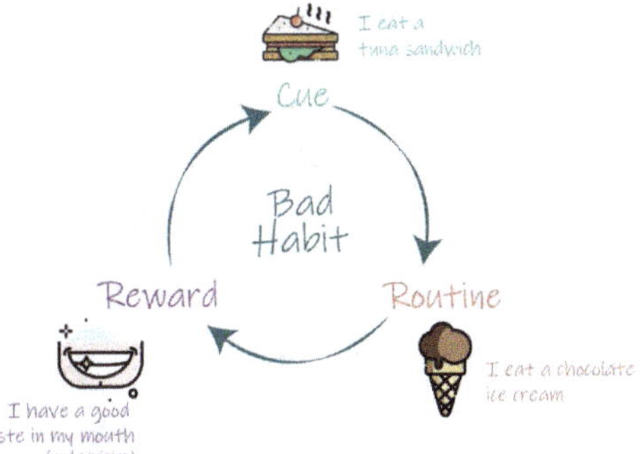

3. Roots of Habit Formation

Energy Conservation: From an evolutionary standpoint, the brain's predilection for habits makes sense. By automating frequent actions, the brain conserves energy, ensuring survival when resources were scarce.

Safety and Efficiency: Habitual behaviours reduced the need for conscious decision-making in familiar situations. Recognising safe paths, known food sources, or routine tasks and automating responses to them ensured both safety and efficiency.

Predictability in an Unpredictable World: Our ancestors lived in a world replete with uncertainties. Habits provided a semblance of predictability and control, establishing routines in daily life that countered external unpredictability.

4. The Dichotomy of Habitual Responses

Adaptive vs. Maladaptive: While habits evolved as adaptive responses, in today's complex world, they can sometimes be maladaptive. For instance, while stress-eating might have been adaptive when food was scarce, it's less so in today's world of plenty, potentially leading to health issues.

Understanding the science behind habits unravels many mysteries of human behaviour. It underscores the fact that we're not just creatures of conscious thought and deliberate action, but also of deeply ingrained patterns sculpted by nature and nurture. This knowledge arms us with the power to mould, modify, and master our habits, aligning them with our aspirations and the spirit of the JFDI philosophy.

Creating Habits that Stick

Establishing a new habit can often feel like trying to carve a path through a dense forest. The initial stages are riddled with resistance, setbacks, and the looming temptation to revert to familiar grounds. However, as with trailblazing, the repeated act of traversing this new path makes it clearer, easier, and more automatic over time. In this segment, we'll explore techniques, strategies, and insights that can guide you in forming habits that not only take root but flourish and endure.

1. The Power of Small Steps

The Two-Minute Rule: James Clear, author of "Atomic Habits", propounds the two-minute rule as a way to initiate a new habit. The premise is simple: start with a version of the habit you can complete in two minutes or less. If you want to read more, begin by reading just one page a night. The idea is to scale the action down so that it's almost ridiculously easy to start.

Compound Growth of Habits: Just as compound interest benefits financial growth; tiny habit increments can lead to significant long-term changes. A 1% improvement every day can lead to a substantial transformation over a year.

2. Consistency Over Intensity

Daily Repetition: A habit is like a muscle—it strengthens with use. Engaging in a desired behaviour daily, even if it's for a short period, ingrains the habit faster than intense, sporadic bursts.

Setting Streaks: Challenge yourself to maintain a streak of consecutive days performing the habit. Apps like "HabitBull" or "Streaks" can help you track and visualise your consistency, offering additional motivation.

Embrace the Plateaus: Every habit journey witnesses plateaus—periods where it feels like no progress is being made. Instead of getting disheartened, recognize plateaus as a natural part of the process and remain steadfast.

3. Anchoring New Habits to Existing Ones

Habit Stacking: Based on the principle of pairing, habit stacking involves integrating a new habit into an existing routine. If you're trying to incorporate mindfulness, for instance, link it to your morning coffee ritual. As you sip, spend a few minutes in quiet reflection or deep breathing.

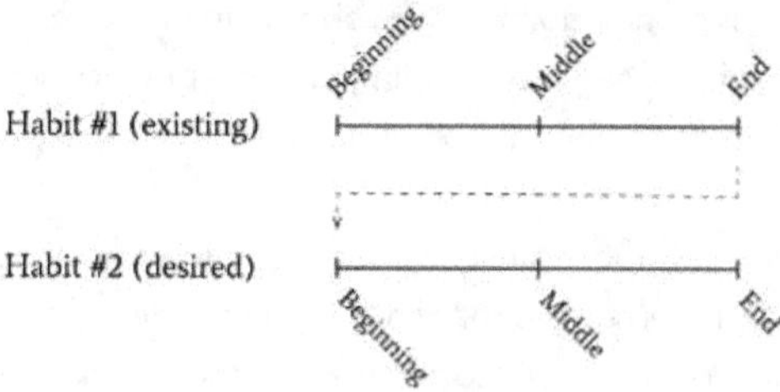

Visual Anchors: Physical reminders can act as powerful anchors. If you're trying to remember to take vitamins, place them beside your toothbrush—a daily-use item. The act of brushing will then prompt the subsequent habit of vitamin consumption.

4. Environment Design for Habit Adherence

Optimising Spaces: Your environment significantly influences behaviour. If you want to cultivate a reading habit, create a cosy reading nook with a comfortable chair, good lighting, and a bookshelf. For fitness enthusiasts, having gym clothes prepared the night before can act as a cue.

Eliminate Friction: Reduce the number of steps between you and your desired habit. If you aim to jog every morning, have your running shoes and outfit ready by your bed.

Minimise Temptations: On the flip side, increase the steps between you and undesirable habits. If you're aiming to reduce screen time, keep your phone in another room during work or sleep hours. Cue the K-Safe!

<u>5. Celebrate Small Wins</u>

Immediate Rewards: While the long-term benefits of habits are evident, the brain responds positively to immediate rewards. After a workout, indulge in a favourite healthy snack. After a meditation session, savour a cup of herbal tea. These instant rewards reinforce the habit loop.

Progress Tracking: Maintain a journal or use habit-tracking apps. Visually seeing your progress acts as a motivator and provides tangible evidence of your commitment.

Affirmations: Positive self-talk and affirmations reinforce belief in oneself. Celebrate your successes, however small, with affirmations like "I am committed to my growth" or "Every step I take is bringing me closer to my goals."

Creating habits that stick is less about grand gestures and more about the daily, consistent, small choices we make. By understanding the mechanics of habit formation and using strategies tailored to human psychology, we can steer our behaviours in directions that align with our goals, values, and the essence of the JFDI philosophy. The road to transformation, after all, is paved with the bricks of habit.

<u>**Daily Rituals for Success**</u>

Across time, many of the world's most successful and influential people have attributed a portion of their accomplishments to their daily rituals. From Benjamin Franklin's structured daily plans to Maya Angelou's solitary writing retreats, rituals create an environment of predictability in the whirlwind of life. But why are these daily rituals so impactful? And more importantly, how can you create your own set of rituals tailored to your aspirations and lifestyle?

<u>1. The Power of Rituals in Anchoring the Day</u>

Setting the Tone: Starting the day with intentionality sets a proactive tone, rather than a reactive one. Whether it's a morning meditation or reviewing the day's tasks over a cup of coffee, these rituals help you mentally prepare and establish a sense of purpose.

Reducing Decision Fatigue: Rituals automate parts of your day. When certain actions become habitual, it frees up mental bandwidth and reduces the fatigue that comes from making too many decisions.

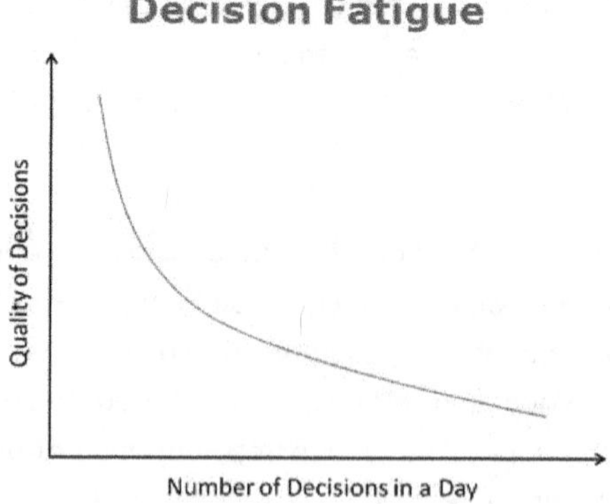

<u>2. Morning Rituals: Harnessing the Fresh Start</u>

Wake Up at a Consistent Time: The body's circadian rhythm thrives on consistency. By waking up at the same time, even on weekends, you regulate your internal clock, leading to better sleep and heightened alertness.

Mindful Movement: Incorporate some form of movement to awaken the body. It could be a full workout, a brief stretching routine, or even a short walk outside. Movement increases blood flow, boosts mood, and enhances cognitive function.

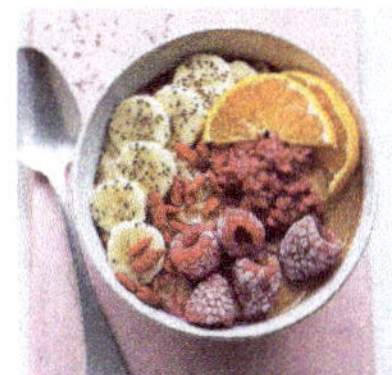

Nourish the Body: A consistent and nutritious breakfast ritual can fuel your body for the tasks ahead. This isn't just about what you eat but also the act of eating itself. Take this time to savour your meal and be present.

Mental Priming: Engage in activities that stimulate the mind and align with your goals. This could be reading, journaling, visualisation exercises, or even reviewing your daily and long-term goals.

<u>3. Midday Rituals: Refocusing and Re-energising</u>

Scheduled Breaks: Taking planned breaks can prevent burnout. Use this time to stretch, take a brief walk, or engage in a short mindfulness exercise.

Nutrition and Hydration: A light, nutritious lunch can prevent the mid-afternoon slump many people experience. Stay hydrated with water or herbal teas to maintain cognitive function.

Mindful Breathing: Just a few minutes of deep breathing can act as a reset button, reducing stress and refocusing the mind.

4. Evening Rituals: Wind Down and Reflect

Digital Detox: Set a specific time each evening to disconnect from digital devices. This reduces blue light exposure, aiding better sleep, and allows the mind to transition from the day's chaos to a more restful state.

Gratitude Practice: Spend a few moments reflecting on the positive aspects of your day. This reinforces a positive mindset and cultivates a habit of seeking out the good.

Preparation for Tomorrow: Set out what you'll need for the next day. This could be choosing an outfit, preparing a to-do list, or setting out workout gear. This simple act reduces morning stress and decision fatigue.

Relaxation Techniques: Engage in activities that signal to your body and mind that it's time to rest. This could be a warm bath, reading, listening to calming music, or a brief meditation session.

5. Creating Your Personalized Ritual

Assess Your Needs and Goals: Everyone's ideal ritual will differ. Some might benefit from a vigorous morning workout, while others might find value in quiet contemplation. Start by understanding what energises you and what aligns with your aspirations.

Stay Flexible: While rituals provide structure, it's essential to remain adaptable. If something isn't serving you or if your circumstances change, tweak your rituals accordingly.

Consistency is Key: Like any habit, the power of rituals lies in their consistent application. Over time, these actions will become second nature, anchoring your day and propelling you towards success.

Daily rituals are more than mere habits; they're sacred routines that bring order to our chaotic lives, creating calm and focus. By grounding ourselves in these rituals, we not only enhance our productivity but also cultivate a deep sense of purpose and mindfulness in our everyday actions. As the JFDI philosophy underscores, it's the daily, intentional steps that lead to monumental success.

The Double-Edged Sword of Habits

Habits, often understood as the automatic behaviours or routines we regularly engage in, possess an incredible power to shape our lives. They're the silent architects of our daily existence, nudging us closer to our dreams or pulling us further away. The duality of habits – their capability to both uplift and hinder – underscores their classification as a double-edged sword.

1. The Constructive Edge: Building Bridges to Success

Automating Positive Actions: The beauty of a good habit lies in its automation. Once established, it acts like a software program running in the background, ensuring we take regular, positive actions with minimal conscious effort.

Compound Effect: Small, positive habits, when repeated consistently, yield compound benefits over time. For instance, reading just 20 minutes daily can translate into multiple books over a year, massively enhancing knowledge and perspective.

Reinforcing Identity: Every time we engage in a positive habit, we are also casting a vote for the person we wish to become. A regular exercise routine doesn't just build muscle or endurance; it strengthens the identity of someone who values health and discipline.

2. The Destructive Edge: Eroding Foundations Unnoticed

Silent Sabotage: Negative habits often operate insidiously. Whether it's mindlessly scrolling through social media or consuming junk food, the immediate repercussions might seem negligible. However, over extended periods, these habits can lead to wasted time, deteriorated health, or missed opportunities.

Cognitive Dissonance: Engaging in behaviours that conflict with our desired self-image can lead to cognitive dissonance—a state of internal conflict. This can erode self-esteem, as there's a mismatch between who we are and who we aspire to be.

Creating Barriers: Bad habits can sometimes act as barriers, preventing the formation of positive ones. For example, the habit of late-night binge-watching can disrupt sleep patterns, making it harder to establish a productive early morning routine.

3. Recognising and Harnessing the Power of Habits

Habit Awareness: Before leveraging the power of habits, one must become aware of their existing routines. Regular reflection and self-assessment can shed light on behaviours that might be operating beneath conscious awareness.

Reframing Habits: It's essential to recognise that not all habits are created equal. What might be a constructive habit for one person (like an evening walk) could be a way of procrastinating for another. The context and individual goals determine a habit's value.

Replacing Rather Than Erasing: Negative habits can't simply be wished away. The neural pathways associated with them have been reinforced over time. The key lies in replacing them with positive alternatives. For example, instead of a sugary snack, one could reach for a piece of fruit.

<u>4. Habit Stacking: Amplifying the Positive Edge</u>

Building on Existing Habits: One effective way to establish a new habit is to stack it onto an existing one. If you already have a routine of having a cup of tea in the morning, use that time to also review your daily tasks.

Consistent Cue, Varied Reward: The brain craves novelty. While the cue for a habit should remain consistent, occasionally varying the reward can increase adherence. For instance, if your exercise routine involves running, occasionally switching up the route can provide a fresh perspective.

Habits, with their dual nature, serve as reminders of the constant choices we make, often subconsciously. By recognising and respecting their power, we can harness their positive edge to build bridges to our aspirations. Conversely, by becoming vigilant of their destructive potential, we can prevent them from eroding our foundations. We must actively choosing habits that propel us forward, while also having the courage to confront and change those that hold us back.

Building a Habit-Driven Environment

If habits are the silent architects of our daily existence, then the environment is the blueprint upon which they're designed. Our surroundings—both physical and digital—greatly influence the habits we form, making it crucial to intentionally craft an environment conducive to positive habits.

<u>1. The Role of Environment in Habit Formation</u>

Immediate Influence: Our immediate environment acts as a continual stream of cues triggering our habits. A visible exercise mat might prompt a morning workout, while a phone notification can send us into a spiral of social media scrolling.

Reinforcing or Disrupting: A well-structured environment can reinforce our desired habits, whereas a chaotic one can disrupt even the most established routines. For example, a tidy workspace can facilitate focused work, while a cluttered one can lead to distraction and procrastination.

2. Crafting the Physical Environment

Strategic Placement: Position items related to positive habits within easy reach. If you're trying to read more, keep a book on your bedside table or coffee table. Conversely, reduce accessibility to distractions or unhealthy temptations by placing them out of sight or making them harder to get to.

Visual Cues: Use visual reminders to prompt desired actions. Post-it notes with motivational quotes, vision boards, or even setting your running shoes next to your bed can serve as nudges towards positive behaviour.

Designated Spaces: Dedicate specific areas for specific activities. Having a particular spot for meditation, reading, or exercise can, over time, make initiating that activity feel automatic when you enter that space.

3. Optimising the Digital Environment

Notification Control: Our devices are a significant source of distraction. Take back control by turning off non-essential notifications. This reduces the number of digital cues pulling you into unproductive or time-wasting habits.

App Organization: Organise apps so that tools for productivity are on your main screen, while potential distractions are tucked away in folders or on secondary pages.

Digital Detox: I hate this term, but regularly schedule periods where you disconnect from digital devices. This not only provides a mental break but can also help in forming habits like reading, outdoor walks, or other non-digital activities.

<u>4. Social Environment and Habits</u>

Power of Association: We often mirror the habits of those around us. Surround yourself with people who embody the habits you wish to adopt. This doesn't mean ditching old friends but intentionally seeking out and spending time with those who inspire growth.

Accountability Partners: Sharing your habit goals with someone can create a mutual system of accountability. Knowing someone will check in on your progress can be a powerful motivator.

Group Activities: Engage in group activities related to your desired habits. Joining a book club, a fitness group, or a hobby class can make habit adoption more enjoyable and sustainable.

Building a habit-driven environment requires a blend of intentionality and consistency. It's about creating a backdrop for your life that continuously nudges you toward better choices. By optimising both physical and digital spaces, and by being mindful of our social environment, we can pave a smoother path towards lasting, positive habit formation. In the journey of self-improvement, our surroundings can be our most powerful ally. It's time we recognise and harness its potential.

Overcoming Habit Plateaus

As we journey on the path of habit formation and personal development, it's common to encounter what many call 'habit plateaus'. These are phases where progress seems to stagnate, motivation wanes, and the vibrant energy that once propelled our routines seems to have ebbed away. Understanding and navigating these plateaus is crucial for sustained growth.

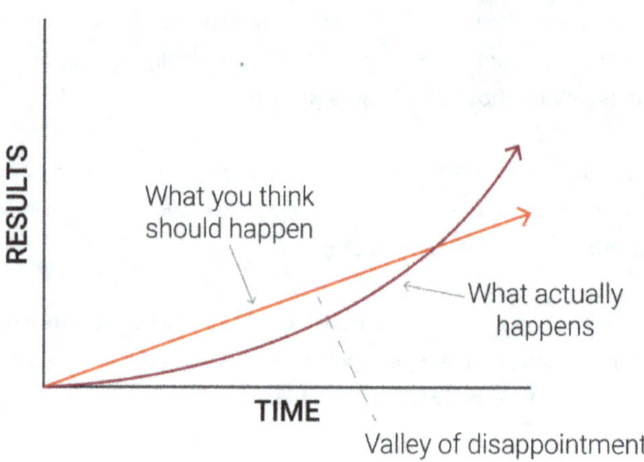

Visual from Atomic Habits by James Clear.

1. Recognising a Habit Plateau

The Subtle Signals: Before addressing a plateau, we must recognise it. Symptoms often include a decline in enthusiasm, a feeling of monotony, or a perceived lack of progress despite consistent effort.

Feedback Mechanisms: Regularly track and review your habits. Using journals, apps, or even simple checklists can help you visually spot when you're hitting a plateau.

2. Understanding the Causes

Natural Progression: Just as in physical fitness, the rapid gains we initially see (or feel) when starting a new habit can slow over time. This is a natural part of progression and doesn't necessarily indicate a failing strategy.

Shifting Motivations: What motivated you at the start of your habit journey might not be what motivates you now. Re-evaluating and understanding your evolving motivations can provide clarity.

Environmental Changes: Sometimes, external changes—like a shift in work schedule, a move to a new place, or personal life events—can disrupt and affect the momentum of our habits.

3. Strategies to Break Through

Re-assess and Re-align: Take a moment to revisit your goals associated with the habit. Are they still relevant? Adjust your habits to align with your current aspirations.

Introduce Variability: Monotony is often a significant contributor to habit plateaus. Introducing small changes or challenges can reinvigorate a stale routine. For instance, if you're used to jogging, try integrating intervals or exploring new routes.

Celebrate Small Wins: Recognize and celebrate the small milestones and progress you've made. This can reignite the motivation and remind you of the growth you've already achieved.

Seek External Input: Sometimes, an external perspective can provide invaluable insights. Whether it's a coach, a friend, or joining a group focused on a similar habit, getting feedback can help identify areas for improvement or adjustment.

<u>4. Leveraging Plateaus for Growth</u>

Embrace the Plateau: Instead of viewing plateaus as setbacks, see them as opportunities for introspection and recalibration. They are natural phases of reflection that allow us to assess and adjust our trajectory.

The Power of Rest: Just as muscles need rest to grow after an intense workout, our brains and willpower can benefit from occasional breaks. Periodic rests can rejuvenate your energy and perspective.

Reconnect with your 'Why': Revisit the core reasons why you started the habit. Reconnecting with your initial inspiration can provide the necessary push to move beyond the plateau.

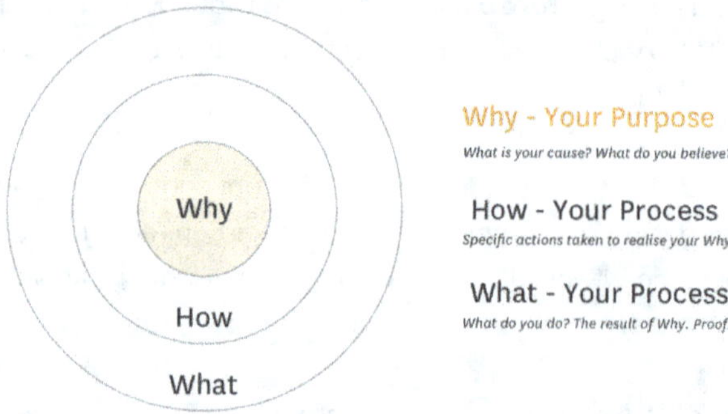

'Start with Why', a talk by Simon Sinek is an excellent resource on discovering your why.

Habit plateaus, though challenging, are an integral part of the growth journey. They test our commitment, resilience, and adaptability. By understanding their nature and deploying effective strategies, we can transform these apparent roadblocks into stepping stones, propelling us even closer to our ultimate goals. Remember, it's not the challenges we face, but how we respond to them, that defines our path forward.

Chapter 10 – Surrounding Yourself with Doers

The Impact of Peer Influence

The adage, "show me your friends, and I'll tell you who you are," has been reiterated across generations, emphasising the undeniable influence peers exert on our behaviours, thoughts, and motivations. Peer influence, for better or worse, can significantly mould our decisions and lifestyle choices. To harness the transformative power of the JFDI philosophy, it's crucial to understand and appreciate how peers impact our journey.

1. The Neuroscience of Peer Influence

Mirror Neurons – Imitation at Play: Deep within the brain lies a special class of neurons known as 'mirror neurons.' These neurons activate both when we perform an action and when we observe someone else do the same. This mirroring mechanism is believed to be foundational for empathy, understanding, and crucially, imitation. When we're around proactive, ambitious individuals, our mirror neurons are more likely to prompt us into similar action, driving us toward accomplishment.

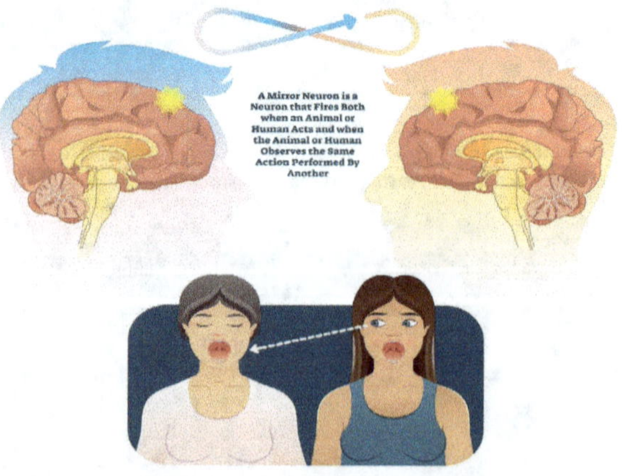

Dopamine and Reward Systems: Social approval and acceptance release dopamine, a neurotransmitter linked to pleasure and motivation. When our peer group values and rewards action, taking steps toward our goals becomes not just a cognitive decision but also a source of neurological reward.

2. The Sociological Dynamics

Conformity and Groupthink: Humans have an innate desire to fit in. We naturally conform to the behaviours, attitudes, and beliefs of our peer group. This phenomenon, known as conformity, ensures social cohesion but can also shape our behaviours. Being part of a group of doers means that proactive behaviours become the 'group norm', making it psychologically easier for members to initiate action.

Status and Social Hierarchies: Within any group, certain behaviours are associated with higher status. If those at the 'top' of a social hierarchy value action, ambition, and achievement, it sets a precedent for others to emulate. Aligning with proactive peers can subconsciously push us to pursue similar pathways to gain status and recognition within the group.

3. Emotional and Motivational Spillover

Shared Energy and Enthusiasm: There's a contagious quality to enthusiasm and energy. When surrounded by motivated individuals who are passionate about their endeavours, we often find our spirits lifted, our reservations diminished, and our drive ignited.

Shared Triumphs and Failures: Being in a circle of doers allows members to celebrate each other's successes and provide support during setbacks. This shared emotional landscape not only reinforces the bond among peers but also offers a safety net, making the journey less daunting.

Online Echo Chambers: In today's interconnected world, our peer group isn't restricted to those we physically interact with. Online communities, forums, and social media amplify peer influence. While these platforms can be empowering, they can also create echo chambers, reinforcing our beliefs and behaviours. Curating our online space to reflect values of proactivity and ambition can have a pronounced effect on our daily actions.

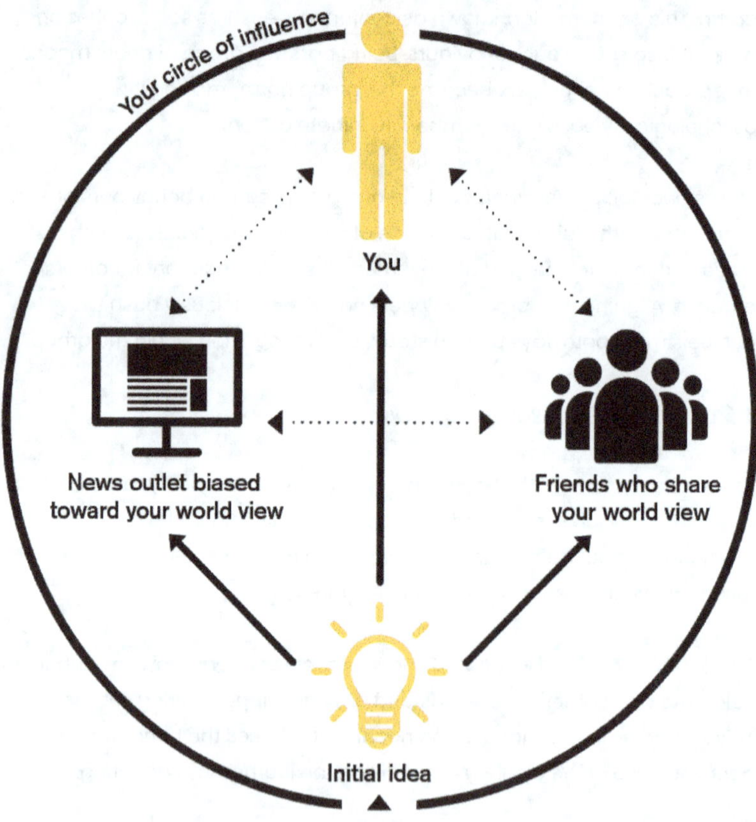

Social Comparison: Digital platforms make it easy to compare our lives with others. While this can inspire and motivate, it can also lead to feelings of inadequacy. It's essential to use these platforms constructively, drawing inspiration from doers while ensuring our self-worth isn't solely tied to online comparisons.

Peer influence is a multifaceted force, shaped by intricate neurological, sociological, and emotional components. Recognising and harnessing this power is pivotal for anyone aiming to embark on the JFDI journey. By intentionally aligning ourselves with doers, we set the stage for positive peer influence to guide, motivate, and propel us toward our goals.

Identifying True Doers

In a world where everyone seems to be chasing success, it's crucial to discern between those who genuinely embody the spirit of "doing" and those who merely project a facade. True doers aren't just about loud declarations and social media updates; they are characterised by consistent actions, resilience, and a growth-oriented mindset. Here's a guide to help you identify, connect with, and learn from these genuine achievers.

1. Beyond the Surface – Substance over Show

Consistency over Intensity: Anyone can have a short burst of motivation or a singular moment of brilliance, but true doers exhibit consistency. Their journey might not always be glamorous, but their unwavering commitment, day in and day out, sets them apart.

Quality of Output: Look beyond frequency and delve into the quality of their work. A true doer is not just active; they are productive and purpose-driven, continually seeking to improve and refine their craft.

<u>2. Values and Ethics</u>

Integrity in Action: True doers maintain their integrity. They're transparent about their methods and don't cut corners or sacrifice their values for short-term gains.

Empathy and Team Spirit: While personal ambition is a driving force, genuine achievers understand the value of teamwork and collaboration. They elevate others, listen with an open heart, and create an environment of mutual respect.

<u>3. Resilience and Adaptability</u>

Facing Failures: Everyone encounters setbacks, but true doers perceive them as learning opportunities. Observe how they navigate challenges and whether they bounce back with renewed vigour and a refined strategy.

Adaptability: In a rapidly changing world, flexibility is a hallmark of a genuine doer. They're not rigidly attached to one path but are agile, ready to pivot and adapt when required, always keeping their ultimate goal in sight.

<u>4. Lifelong Learning</u>

Curiosity: True doers possess an insatiable curiosity. They're always keen to learn, whether it's mastering a new skill, exploring a novel idea, or understanding different perspectives.

Mentorship and Guidance: Genuine achievers recognize that growth is mutual. They actively seek mentorship and, in turn, are willing to guide and nurture upcoming talents, fostering a cycle of continuous learning.

5. Authenticity and Authentic Connections

Real-world Relationships: While online presence can offer insights, nothing beats real-world interactions to gauge authenticity. Engage in conversations, attend events or workshops they might be hosting, and observe their interactions with others.

Consistent Narrative: Their actions, words, and values align. True doers have a congruence in what they say and what they do, both online and offline.

6. Self-awareness and Reflection

Growth from Reflection: Genuine achievers regularly introspect. They're aware of their strengths and weaknesses and constantly work towards self-improvement, not just in their professional endeavours but in personal growth as well.

Accepting Feedback: A hallmark of a true doer is their openness to feedback. They appreciate constructive criticism and use it as a tool to better themselves.

Identifying true doers is an art of observation, engagement, and discernment. Surrounding oneself with such individuals can profoundly influence our journey, infusing it with inspiration, genuine guidance, and a spirit of relentless pursuit. Remember, it's not the noise that defines a doer, but the harmonious symphony of consistent actions, values, and growth.

Finding Your Tribe

Your tribe — the group of individuals you choose to surround yourself with — plays a pivotal role in shaping your mindset, values, behaviours, and ultimately, your success. This section delves into the significance of building your tribe and offers guidance on how to thoughtfully curate this circle of influence.

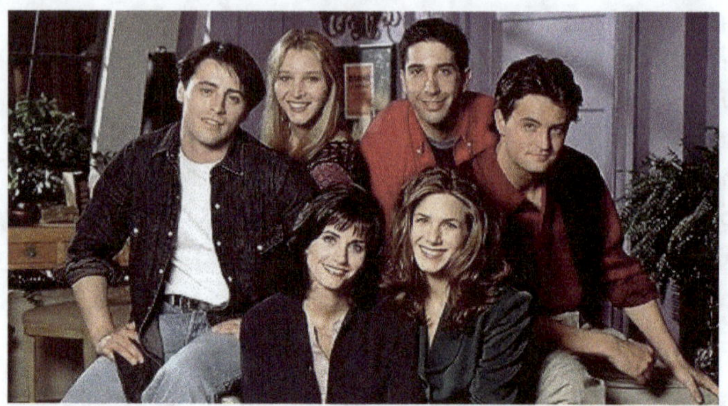

1. Recognizing the Power of a Tribe

Shared Values and Beliefs: At the core of any tribe is a shared set of values and beliefs. This common ground fosters mutual understanding, collaboration, and encouragement, allowing members to propel each other forward.

Collective Momentum: While individual determination is potent, the collective energy of a tribe amplifies motivation, turning individual sparks into a roaring blaze of progress and achievement.

2. The Quest for Quality over Quantity

Depth over Breadth: It's crucial to prioritize the depth of connections over the sheer number. A smaller group of genuinely supportive and aligned individuals can be far more impactful than a vast network of superficial contacts.

Mutual Growth: Seek out individuals who are as invested in your growth as they are in their own. The best tribes consist of members who lift each other up, challenge each other, and celebrate each other's victories.

3. Diversifying Your Tribe

Mix of Expertise: Surrounding yourself with individuals from diverse fields can offer fresh perspectives, inspire creativity, and open doors to opportunities you might not have considered.

Balancing Experience: While it's beneficial to have seasoned veterans in your tribe, it's equally valuable to include newcomers who bring fresh energy, novel ideas, and a different outlook on challenges.

4. Actively Seeking Your Tribe

Networking Events and Workshops: Actively attend industry-specific events, seminars, and workshops. Such platforms are teeming with like-minded individuals, potential mentors, and future collaborators.

Online Communities: Digital platforms and social media groups centered around specific interests, professions, or goals can be goldmines for finding tribe members. Engage actively, contribute value, and build genuine connections.

Recommendations: Leverage your existing network to identify potential tribe members. Personal introductions and recommendations often lead to deeper, more meaningful connections.

5. Nurturing Tribe Relationships

Consistent Engagement: Building a tribe isn't a one-time activity. Consistent engagement, through meet-ups, brainstorming sessions, or just casual catch-ups, strengthens bonds and ensures the tribe's energy remains vibrant.

Give and Take: Ensure that the relationship is mutual. As much as you seek guidance, support, and resources, be prepared to offer the same in return. This reciprocity ensures the tribe thrives.

6. Evolving with Your Tribe

Ebb and Flow: As you grow and evolve, so will your tribe. Members might come and go, and that's natural. The key is to continuously align with those who resonate with your current goals and aspirations.

Ongoing Assessment: Regularly take a step back and assess the value and alignment of your tribe. Ensure that the collective energy remains positive, supportive, and growth-oriented.

Finding your tribe isn't just about surrounding yourself with people. It's about curating a circle that amplifies your strengths, bolsters your weaknesses, and relentlessly pushes you towards your dreams. It's an ongoing journey of alignment, growth, and mutual elevation. Remember, in the world of personal and professional development, your tribe doesn't just signify where you belong — it profoundly impacts where you're headed.

Mentors and Role Models

In a world teeming with ambition and visions, sometimes the most decisive catalyst for our progress is the guidance and inspiration from those who have paved the way before us. Mentors and role models serve as beacons, illuminating the path forward, helping us avoid pitfalls, and offering a compass when we feel lost. This section delves deeply into the invaluable roles these figures play in our journeys and provides insights on how to seek, connect with, and learn from them.

1. Understanding the Difference: Mentors vs. Role Models

Mentors: These are individuals with whom you have a direct, personal relationship. They offer tailored advice, feedback, and guidance based on their experiences and insights. They're invested in your growth, and they provide hands-on support throughout your journey.

Role Models: Often, these are individuals you may never meet. They might be industry leaders, renowned personalities, or even fictional characters. Their life stories, philosophies, and achievements provide a template or source of inspiration for your aspirations.

2. The Impact of Mentors and Role Models

Shortening the Learning Curve: With their experience, mentors can guide you around mistakes they've made or seen, providing shortcuts to success and ensuring efficient progress.

Inspiration and Motivation: The achievements and mindset of role models can serve as a constant source of inspiration. Their stories remind us of what's possible and fuel our drive.

Networking Opportunities: Mentors often introduce their mentees to their professional networks, opening doors to opportunities and connections that can be transformative.

3. Seeking the Right Mentors

Alignment with Goals: Ensure that potential mentors resonate with your current goals and visions. Their experiences and insights should be relevant to the path you're on.

Openness to Mentorship: Not all experienced individuals are open to or suitable for mentorship. Seek those who exhibit a genuine interest in guiding others.

Diversity of Thought: Consider mentors from diverse backgrounds, industries, or disciplines. They can offer fresh perspectives and challenge your thinking in constructive ways.

4. Drawing Inspiration from Role Models

Study Their Journey: Dive deep into their life stories, challenges, and turning points. Understand the mindset shifts and strategies they employed to overcome obstacles.

Emulate, Don't Imitate: While it's beneficial to draw lessons from role models, it's essential to adapt their strategies to your unique situation rather than copying them verbatim.

Stay Updated: If your role models are contemporary figures, follow their ongoing work, writings, and interviews. Their evolution can offer continuous insights and lessons.

5. Building and Nurturing the Relationship with Mentors

Initiate with Clarity: When reaching out to potential mentors, be clear about why you seek their guidance and what you hope to achieve from the mentorship.

Regular Check-ins: Schedule consistent meetings or check-ins. This ensures you remain on track and allows the mentor to provide timely advice.

Reciprocity: While mentorship often leans on the mentor's experience, it's a two-way street. Find ways to offer value back, whether through your unique skills, fresh insights, or simply gratitude and acknowledgment.

6. Evolving with Your Mentors and Role Models

Reassess and Realign: As you grow, your needs from a mentor might evolve. It's okay to seek new mentors who align with your current phase.

Transitioning from Role Models to Peers: There may come a time when individuals you once saw as distant role models become peers or collaborators. Embrace these moments as signs of your growth.

Mentors and role models are more than just figures of admiration or guidance. They are lighthouses in our personal and professional storms, guiding us towards shores of success, fulfilment, and achievement. Embracing their influence, learning from their journeys, and forging genuine connections can significantly amplify our trajectories in the relentless pursuit of our dreams.

Outro

As we approach the end of this transformative journey, it's time to step back, reflect, and understand the power of the philosophy we've delved into: **Just Fucking Do It**.

Throughout this book, we've dismantled barriers, dived deep into our psyches, confronted our fears, and celebrated the beauty of momentum. However, the crux of it all is incredibly simple: start where you are, use what you have, and do what you can.

Procrastination, doubts, and fear of failure are inherent aspects of the human experience. But as we've learned, they're not insurmountable. When faced with the paralysis of overthinking, the most potent antidote is action—no matter how small. It's not about awaiting perfection but about embracing imperfection as a part of the growth journey.

Remember, the world is brimming with ideas, but it's those who act upon them who leave an indelible mark. Every individual with success, from industry disruptors like Airbnb's founders to the relentless passion of Colonel Sanders and Sarah Blakely, began with a simple step, an action, a commitment to bringing their vision to life.

So, as you close this book and venture out into the world with a renewed mindset, remember this: time will pass regardless. It's the choices we make and the actions we take daily that determine our legacies.

It's easy to dream, wish, and hope. But to achieve? That requires the grit to JFDI.

Thank you for embarking on this journey. Now, it's your turn. Take your aspirations, mesh them with the principles you've learned, and step into the world ready to JFDI.

Here's to a future of unwavering action, relentless pursuit, and unforgettable impact. Carry the JFDI torch forward, and light the way for others to follow.

The future depends on what you do today.

Dare to do. Dare to achieve. Just F**king Do It.

www.ingramcontent.com/pod-product-compliance
Lightning Source LLC
Chambersburg PA
CBHW060756260726
48660CB00002B/644